Virtual Reality Interventions for Patients under Palliative Care

Virtual Reality Interventions for Patients under Palliative Care is a groundbreaking guide that empowers healthcare professionals to transform end-of-life care with the innovative use of virtual reality (VR).

This book equips clinicians with the knowledge and skills they need to seamlessly integrate state-of-the-art VR technology into palliative care, addressing a wide range of patient needs, from pain management to wish fulfillment. The book's special features include evidence-based VR interventions, practical implementation strategies, assessment tools, case studies, clinical tips, and suggested scripts for engagement, preparation, and assessment.

Grounded in robust research, theory, and practical expertise, this guidebook is a must-read for any researcher or professional who wants to enhance the quality of life for terminally ill patients and their families through VR technology, which offers a novel and transformative approach that sets it apart from traditional palliative care practices.

Olive K. L. Woo is a licensed clinical psychologist, certified thanatologist, and the founder of Flourishing-Life-Of-Wish Virtual Reality Therapy (FLOW-VRT ®).

W0234821

"This book offers a wealth of research-informed approaches to applying virtual reality technology in palliative care. It provides a valuable blend of scientific insights and clinical breakthroughs. Every healthcare professional and academic researcher will want to have it on their office bookshelf."

Huang Yu-Te, PhD, *associate professor, Department of Social Work and Social Administration, the University of Hong Kong*

"Virtual Reality Interventions for Patients under Palliative Care is a unique and valuable guide for palliative care professionals. Dr. Olive Woo describes how virtual reality can help patients with terminal illness reduce symptoms and improve quality of life. The book describes how to use virtual reality to give patients a sense of joy, closure, and a meaningful end-of-life experience."

Elizabeth McMahon, PhD, *author of* Virtual Reality Therapy for Anxiety: A Guide for Therapists

Virtual Reality Interventions for Patients under Palliative Care

A Practical Guide for Healthcare Professionals

Olive K. L. Woo

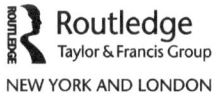

Routledge
Taylor & Francis Group

NEW YORK AND LONDON

Designed cover image: Getty Images

First published 2026
by Routledge
605 Third Avenue, New York, NY 10158

and by Routledge
4 Park Square, Milton Park, Abingdon, Oxon, OX14 4RN

Routledge is an imprint of the Taylor & Francis Group, an informa business

ISBN: 978-1-032-85469-4 (hbk)
ISBN: 978-1-032-85467-0 (pbk)
ISBN: 978-1-003-51832-7 (ebk)

DOI: 10.4324/9781003518327

Typeset in Galliard
by Apex CoVantage, LLC

For my parents, whose unconditional love has not only shaped me but also inspired me to extend that love to those in need.

Contents

Acknowledgements

I am deeply grateful to the many individuals who have contributed to the completion of this book. Their support, guidance, and invaluable insights have been instrumental in shaping this work.

First and foremost, I would like to express my heartfelt appreciation to Dr. Mike Wong, who has supported my exploration of using virtual reality in clinical settings, and Dr. Jeffrey Liu, who has given me unfailing support since the first day of my life journey as a clinical psychologist. Their unwavering dedication to patient care has been a constant source of inspiration and guidance.

I am particularly grateful to my dear mentor and academic supervisor, Dr. Antoinette Lee, for her unwavering support and guidance during my doctoral research on the use of virtual reality in palliative care settings, which ultimately inspired the creation of this book. With her professional assistance, we developed an evidence-based VR-powered psychological intervention named Flourishing-Life-Of-Wish Virtual Reality Therapy (FLOW-VRT®). Her expertise and mentorship have been invaluable in shaping my academic and professional journey.

I would also like to express my deepest gratitude to my colleague, Dr. Gloria Chan, for her constructive feedback on the chapter on skills development. Her keen eye for detail, clinical experiences, and thoughtful suggestions have been invaluable in refining and improving the content.

I am also indebted to Ms. Wing Yen Oh, Mr. Hoi Ho Kong and Ms. Pui Chin Kwok for their diligent efforts in assisting with the literature search.

I would also like to express my deepest gratitude to my parents, who have supported me unconditionally and allowed me to pursue my passion and dreams, one of which is the creation of this book.

Finally, I am thankful to the reviewers who provided constructive feedback during the review process. Their insights have helped to improve the clarity, depth, and overall quality of this book.

To all those who have contributed to this book, I am truly grateful. Your support, expertise, and dedication have been instrumental in bringing this work to fruition.

About the Author

Dr Olive K. L. Woo, PsyD, is a licensed clinical psychologist with over a decade of clinical experiences in public settings. She is a fellow in Thanatology with the Association of Death Education and Counselling in the USA. She has been serving as Honorary Clinical Supervisor at both the University of Hong Kong and the Chinese University of Hong Kong, where she contributes her expertise to the development of future psychologists.

Olive has delivered virtual reality-assisted interventions to over 500 individuals under palliative care since 2020. She is the founder of the evidence-based psychological intervention titled Flourishing-Life-Of-Wish-Virtual Reality Therapy (FLOW-VRT®), which she developed specifically for palliative care. She has authored peer-reviewed publications and has gained media coverage for her research work. Relevant teaching experience includes guest speaking at the University of Hong Kong.

Preface

In the quiet moments of my early career as a clinical psychologist and thanatologist, I was struck by the raw humanity of the last wishes expressed by patients nearing the end of their lives. These were not complex or unattainable dreams but simple, heartfelt desires—like the wish to return home or witness the aurora borealis. These requests resonated deeply within me, underscoring the human need for connection, joy, and closure, even in the face of mortality. Yet, despite my training and dedication, I often felt powerless to help bring these dreams to life.

It was this sense of limitation that propelled me to seek out innovative ways to meet the unmet needs of my patients. My journey led me to the transformative potential of virtual reality (VR) technology. With VR, I discovered that even the most physically confined patients could be transported to distant places and cherished memories. I watched as individuals, bound to their beds for weeks or months, explored the North Pole, climbed mountains, or strolled through home villages—all through the immersive power of VR. These experiences brought smiles to their faces, eased their suffering, and gave them moments of true presence in a world beyond their physical limitations.

Over time, my clinical experiences were further reinforced by a growing body of evidence supporting the use of VR in palliative care. Recent systematic reviews have reported its potential to alleviate pain, reduce anxiety, and improve emotional well-being in patients facing terminal illnesses. Research highlights how immersive environments can address not only physical symptoms but also the psychological, social, and spiritual needs of patients. This evidence, combined with my personal observations, affirmed the immense potential of VR as a therapeutic tool to enhance the quality of end-of-life care.

This book, *Virtual Reality Interventions for Patients under Palliative Care: A Practical Guide for Healthcare Professionals*, reflects the lessons I have learned on a journey of discovery and innovation, shaped by a deep commitment to improving the lives of those at their most vulnerable moments. In addition to sharing my own experiences, this book presents the latest research and highlights global efforts to establish VR as an evidence-based approach in palliative care. It is my hope that this guide will offer both inspiration and practical support to healthcare professionals who wish to incorporate VR technology into their practice, making the impossible possible.

In the following pages, you will find a detailed exploration of the theoretical foundations, practical applications, and ethical considerations of using VR in palliative care. From managing pain to fulfilling end-of-life wishes, this book offers evidence-based interventions and case examples to help you harness the power of VR in ways that are meaningful and compassionate.

As you read, I encourage you to reflect on the profound impact that even small moments of joy, connection, and presence can have on a patient's journey. I hope this book inspires you to explore new ways to support our patients and reminds you of the immense potential we have, as healthcare professionals to make a difference.

Ultimately, this book is not just about technology—it is about humanity. It is about finding ways to bring light to the darkest moments, to offer comfort where there is pain, and to help our patients flourish, even as they approach life's end.

May this guide empower you to create those moments of light.

Olive
July 2025

Introduction

My Story

"I wish to see the aurora borealis."

When I first delivered psychological services to patients[1] with terminal illnesses, I was constantly reminded of the poignant last wishes they expressed. Over and over again, I heard them share their last wishes to travel to their dream destinations, such as the aurora borealis; a wish that resonated deeply within me. After all, if I were in their shoes, I too would want to spend my final days in a comforting or familiar place rather than confined to a bed. The frustration of feeling limited in what I could do, as a clinical psychologist and thanatologist, to help them fulfil their last wishes drove me to explore alternative methods that could help make the impossible possible. It was during this quest that I discovered the incredible potential of virtual reality (VR). I realized that this technology could offer patients an opportunity to visit any place they wish, in a virtual, but yet fulfilling way.

From that moment on, I make it my mission to incorporate VR into my routine psychological services. I work tirelessly to study the palliative care literature, gather resources, and establish collaboration with multidisciplinary professionals in palliative care to deliver VR interventions to patients at their end-of-life stage. Their response has been awe-inspiring. As patients immerse themselves in the virtual world, I witness remarkable transformations unfold before my eyes. Their physical and emotional symptoms begin to improve. Those who had been bedridden for weeks or even months were suddenly able to explore the sandy shores of a tropical beach, climb majestic mountains, or stroll through bustling city streets. Thanks to the immersive nature of VR, patients can experience a sense of *presence* (Minsky, 1980), feeling as if they are "being there" in the virtual environment, such as marvelling at the aurora borealis at the North Pole, even while physically confined to their beds.

DOI: 10.4324/9781003518327-1

Witnessing the positive impact of VR on patients' lives fuelled my determination to expand the application of VR further. Under Dr Antoinette Lee's supervision, I developed a novel psychological intervention named Flourishing-Life-Of-Wish Virtual Reality Therapy (FLOW-VRT®), which was specifically designed to improve the quality of end-of-life care by alleviating physical and emotional distress. FLOW-VRT is founded on flow (Csikszentmihalyi, 1975), attention restoration (Kaplan, 1995, 2001), self-determination (Deci & Ryan, 2000), and stress coping theory (Lazarus & Folkman, 1984). I named the therapy "Flourishing-Life-Of-Wish" (FLOW), to highlight that this intervention can help fulfil the wishes of patients approaching death, and help them "flourish." In positive psychology, the concept of "flourishing" refers to a state of optimal well-being and fulfilment, where individuals experience positive emotions, engage in meaningful activities, and have a sense of purpose and accomplishment. I believe that even when patients are approaching death, they can still flourish with a sense of joy, closure, and a rewarding experience. They may even experience *flow*, a psychological state characterized by a deep sense of engagement, enjoyment, and immersion in an activity (Engeser et al., 2021). As the principal investigator of the research team, our randomized controlled trial observed a significant decrease in palliative symptoms in the specialized version of FLOW-VRT known as "FLOW-VRT-Relaxation" when compared to the conventional relaxation methods used in palliative care settings (Woo et al., 2024).

Why I Wrote This Book

Writing this book has been my dream. I hope to share all my clinical experiences and knowledge regarding the use of VR interventions for patients at their end-of-life stage. As a healthcare professional who has witnessed the radiant smiles in tetraplegic or bedbound patients after the immersive power of VR, I want to offer my research as an exemplar to indicate that as long as we have the heart for patient benefit, we can always bring something helpful or special to patients. I want as many patients as possible to benefit from VR-assisted interventions, and I want many therapists like me to have a sense of fulfilment when they witness patients' joyful smiles and alleviated symptoms after VR, gained through wish fulfilment and less suffering.

This book aims to prepare you, my dear reader, for the efficacious delivery of VR interventions. I hope to provide the relevant knowledge, skills, and attitudes required for the quality delivery of such interventions. To the best of my knowledge, there is regrettably no dedicated, comprehensive text or guidebook on the topic of applying VR technologies in palliative care settings. This gap in the literature has made it challenging for clinicians to access the necessary information, resources, and guidance to confidently and responsibly incorporate these emerging interventions into their practice. This has motivated me to author this book, which hopefully, will fill this void and empower healthcare professionals across different disciplines to leverage the therapeutic benefits of VR interventions to support our vulnerable patients. My individual reach and resources are inherently limited. However, I hope that by sharing my clinical experiences and knowledge through this book, I can amplify the dissemination of VR interventions so that a greater number of patients in need of palliative care can access and benefit from the potential of these technologies to alleviate their suffering and improve their overall well-being.

Purpose of the Book

I wrote this book to provide aspiring clinicians with a comprehensive guide on the therapeutic use of VR for patients with terminal illnesses. It is the first of its kind to focus specifically on the clinical application of VR in palliative care, taking into account the growing body of scientific evidence supporting its clinical efficacy. This book covers a wide range of topics, including the theoretical foundations for the use of VR, its practical implementation, and ethical considerations. It details a wide range of applications for VR, which include but are not limited to pain management, wish fulfilment, relaxation practice, and reminiscence. The intended audience for this book includes psychologists, social workers, counsellors, researchers, and graduates with a background in thanatology, palliative care, psychology, nursing, VR, and related fields. The book caters to both beginners who seek to explore the clinical use of VR in palliative care and experienced professionals looking to enhance their clinical skills and knowledge of this innovative tool.

The purpose of this guide is to help you:

- Understand palliative care in terms of its basic principles, the patient's specific and unmet needs, and traditional psychological interventions.
- Understand VR and its applications, research, and possible theoretical foundations in palliative care.
- Understand the clinical applications of VR in palliative care that address the physical, psychological, social, and spiritual needs of patients, as well as the training and psychological needs of palliative care providers.
- Be aware of the ethical considerations involved in using VR in palliative care, including the potential physical and psychological risks and the training required for a VR facilitator.

- Understand the future research and clinical directions of using VR in palliative care.
- Learn how VR works in clinical practice based on evidence-based support and multiple case examples.
- Integrate VR with interventions in various treatment modules, such as cognitive behavioural therapy and music therapy.

About Virtual Reality and Patient Responses

VR is a technology that uses computer systems to create simulated environments. Its specialized equipment includes a head-mounted device and controllers, which allow users to interact with the virtual environment. VR is able to integrate visual graphics with multiple sensory cues to create an evocative environment (Gerardi et al., 2010, 2008). Such simulations can trigger psychological, emotional, and physical responses, such as joy, anxiety, and sweating, which are similar to real-life reactions (Martens et al., 2019). With such characteristics, VR has been regarded as a potentially revolutionary tool for the psychological treatment of various mental disorders (Freeman et al., 2017).

Most patients who are willing to try VR give positive feedback after using the technology in palliative care settings. It is not uncommon to witness patients' joy, excitement, and gratitude when they experience VR for the first time. Some participants express a sense of awe and wonder as they immerse themselves in virtual environments and engage in activities they previously thought were impossible. They are often amazed at how "realistic" the virtual environment looks to them and they feel a heightened sense of presence and connection to the virtual world. I witness one patient who was highly appreciative of her virtual travel under the deep sea, where she could swim with the fishes and sea tortoises when she was bedbound with a nasal cannula and stoma bag. She shared that she always wanted to dive deep into the sea but was too afraid to do so in real life.

However, some patients may initially reject the use of VR, as they may not perceive it as being helpful or relevant to their situation. This can be especially true for patients who are experiencing low mood, a low sense of acceptance towards their palliative status, or significant physical constraints, such as feeling too tired or experiencing dizziness. In such cases, it is important to take a cautious and ethical approach to the delivery of VR interventions, ranging from screening suitable patients to debriefing the VR session. This book provides practical suggestions on the thorough ethical and quality delivery of VR interventions and the potential psychological and physical risks associated with the use of VR in palliative care.

Special Features of the Book

Evidence-Based Virtual Reality Interventions

This guidebook presents various VR applications in palliative care that address the physical, psychological, social, and spiritual needs of patients at their end-of-life stage. It provides information on specific VR interventions that have been studied and shown to be efficacious in the therapeutic contexts of palliative care.

Practical Implementation Strategies

This guidebook offers a unique feature of providing practical implementation strategies to accompany VR interventions. It also offers practical tips for inviting patients to try this novel intervention, with elaborations on possible patient responses, preparing patients for VR interventions, ensuring patient comfort, and managing potential risks such as cybersickness or emotional distress. It also includes troubleshooting tips and suggestions for creating a safe and comfortable VR environment for patients at the end-of-life stage.

Integration of Theory and Practice

This guidebook goes beyond providing practical instructions and techniques. As VR intervention in palliative care is an emerging field, the guidebook examines its possible theoretical foundations by exploring related psychological theories, such as self-determination, flow, restoration, and stress–coping theory. It also explores essential concepts, such as the sense of presence. The guidebook also provides insight into integrating various theories into clinical practices, ensuring a holistic and theoretically grounded approach to patient care.

Assessment Tools

This guidebook suggests assessment methods and tools for integrating VR interventions into palliative care that help clinicians gather comprehensive information about patients and their presenting concerns. The assessment tool allows clinicians to evaluate patients' biopsychosocial–spiritual needs and the potential risks associated with VR interventions. These tools range from reviewing medical records to collecting outcome data to facilitate thorough assessment and treatment planning.

Case Studies

This guidebook is supplemented with case studies that demonstrate the application of VR interventions. These real-life scenarios hopefully provide clinicians with practical insights and inspiration on how to effectively incorporate VR interventions into their palliative care practice. The case studies showcase the diverse applications of VR interventions; for example, in addressing unresolved pain, unfulfilled wishes, and unmet emotional needs.

Clinical Pearls

Clinical pearls throughout this guidebook offer valuable insights, practical tips, therapeutic techniques, and troubleshooting based on the scientific literature and my clinical experiences and knowledge. The guidebook also includes guidance on addressing patients' emotional discomfort and optimizing the therapeutic process with VR interventions. It also provides practical solutions and suggestions for the common challenges that healthcare professionals may encounter when using VR in palliative care.

Note

1 The term "patient" is used throughout this book to refer to individuals in need of palliative care and the potential recipients of virtual reality interventions in settings such as care homes for older adults, community centers, hospices, hostels, and individual residences.

References

Csikszentmihalyi, M. (1975). *Beyond boredom and anxiety.* Jossey-Bass Publishers.
Deci, E. L., & Ryan, R. M. (2000). The "what" and "why" of goal pursuits: Human needs and the self-determination of behavior. *Psychological Inquiry, 11,* 227–268.
Engeser, S., Schiepe-Tiska, A., & Peifer, C. (2021). Historical lines and an overview of current research on flow. In *Advances in flow research* (pp. 1–29). Springer International Publishing. https://doi.org/10.1007/978-3-030-53468-4_1
Freeman, D., Reeve, S., Robinson, A., Ehlers, A., Clark, D., Spanlang, B., & Slater, M. (2017). Virtual reality in the assessment, understanding, and treatment of mental health disorders. *Psychological Medicine, 47*(14), 2393–2400. https://doi.org/10.1017/S003329171700040X
Gerardi, M., Cukor, J., Difede, J., Rizzo, A., & Rothbaum, B. (2010). Virtual reality exposure therapy for post-traumatic stress disorder and other anxiety disorders. *Current Psychiatry Reports, 12,* 298–305.
Gerardi, M., Rothbaum, B., Ressler, K., Heekin, M., & Rizzo, A. (2008). Virtual reality exposure therapy using a virtual Iraq: Case report. *Journal of Traumatic Stress, 21,* 209–213.
Kaplan, S. (1995). The restorative benefits of nature: Toward an integrative framework. *Journal of Environmental Psychology, 15,* 169–182.

Kaplan, S. (2001). Meditation, restoration and the management of mental fatigue. *Environment and Behaviour, 33*, 480–506.

Lazarus, R. S., & Folkman, S. (1984). *Stress, appraisal and coping*. Springer.

Martens, M. A., Antley, A., Freeman, D., Slater, M., Harrison, P. J., & Tunbridge, E. M. (2019). It feels real: Physiological responses to a stressful virtual reality environment and its impact on working memory. *Journal of Psychopharmacology (Oxford), 33*(10), 1264–1273. https://doi.org/10.1177/0269881119860156

Minsky, M. (1980). *Telepresence* (pp. 45–51). Omni.

Woo, O. K. L., Lee, A. M., Ng, R., Eckhoff, D., Lo, R., & Cassinelli, A. (2024). Flourishing-Life-Of-Wish Virtual Reality Therapy (FLOW-VRT-Relaxation) outperforms traditional relaxation therapy in palliative care: Results from a randomized controlled trial. *Frontiers in Virtual Reality, 4*. https://doi.org/10.3389/frvir.2023.1304155

Section I

Overview of Palliative Care

This section provides a comprehensive overview of palliative care that lays the foundation of VR interventions by explaining the fundamental principles, goals, and philosophy of palliative care. Chapter 1 provides an introduction to the field of palliative care and discusses the specific needs of patients in this context, Chapter 2 elaborates on the traditional psychological interventions employed in palliative care, and Chapter 3 highlights the unmet needs that still exist within the clinical field.

DOI: 10.4324/9781003518327-2

1 Understanding Palliative Care
Background and Specific Patient Needs

Introduction

In the realm of palliative care, where every moment is precious, the focus shifts to more than just symptom management—it becomes a journey of compassion, dignity, and care. This chapter sets the foundation for understanding palliative care and, in later chapters, how virtual reality (VR) can transform this landscape, offering hope and connection to those facing terminal illnesses. The chapter covers a brief background of palliative care and the specific needs of patients with terminal illnesses. It introduces the importance of patient-centred approach and presents the biopsychosocial-spiritual model (Sulmasy, 2002) that highlights a comprehensive framework for understanding and addressing the multifaceted needs of patients at their end-of-life stage. A task-based model (Corr, 1992) is further discussed as a practical framework for organizing and delivering palliative care interventions. Supportive Care Framework for Cancer Care (Fitch, 2008) is elaborated to facilitate further understanding of supportive care for patients with cancer.

Palliative Care

"There is an end of cure; there is no end of care."

(Verma, 2018)

Derived from the Latin word "pallium," "palliative" means to cloak or cover up, i.e., to alleviate symptoms of illnesses without curing them. The philosophical underpinning of palliative care is to maximize an individual's quality of life by managing physical symptoms while providing psychological, social, and spiritual support. Palliative care is later defined by the World Health Organization (2023) as an "approach that improves the quality of life of patients—adults and children—and their families who are facing

DOI: 10.4324/9781003518327-3

problems associated with life-threatening illness." It was cited that an estimated 4.4 million people in the WHO European Region, including 140 00 children, need palliative care each year (World Health Organization, 2023). Palliative care is advised to be available in hospitals, palliative care units, hospices, and in primary care through home care teams. The need for palliative care is expected to grow in view of the ageing population and the increasing incidence of noncommunicable diseases.

Patient-Centred Care

Patient-centred care has been recognized as a benchmark of supportive care for patients with terminal illnesses (Department of Health, 2000; Institute of Medicine, 2001). It emphasizes support that caters to an individual's needs, preferences, and values (Mead & Bower, 2000), while individual needs are often multifaceted (Asadi-Lari et al., 2004). Particularly in cancer care, medical treatments often have uncertain outcomes that warrant weighting of benefit and cost for individual patients (Butow & Tattersall, 2005) that caters to individual needs and preferences (Epstein & Street, 2007). Such an optimal patient-centred approach aims to maximize health outcomes, ultimately improving the quality of end-of-life care (Stewart, 1995).

Biopsychosocial-Spiritual Model

Biopsychosocial-spiritual model provides a framework that advocates a holistic approach in supporting patients under palliative care. It is rooted in the biopsychosocial model, which was first brought to medicine by Engel (1978, 2012), who highlighted that every healthcare task should address the biological, psychological, and social aspects of an individual. It is a model that helps philosophical understanding of how the illness may be affected by societal factors and practical understanding that an individual's subjective experience relates to health and humane care (Borrell-Carrió et al., 2004). The spiritual dimension is later added to for a more thorough understanding of health outcomes (Katerndahl, 2008). With the spiritual element, the biopsychosocial–spiritual model is justified to be a more comprehensive model of care by addressing the totality of the patient's relational existence (Sulmasy, 2002). Aligned with the patient-centred and holistic approach, the biopsychosocial-spiritual model has been widely adopted among patients with terminal illnesses (Beng, 2004; Sulmasy, 2002).

Task-Based Model

Another framework that has been widely adopted in palliative care is the task-based model (Corr, 1992). It identifies four tasks that patient at their end-of-life stage can play an active role in performing for enhanced quality of life. Aligned with the aforementioned biopsychosocial-spiritual model, the task-based model has the physical, psychological, social, and spiritual dimensions. A patient is suggested to approach death as an actor, instead of a reactor, who can act according to an individual's preferences and values. Such a task-based approach provides a benchmark that helps identify life regrets and act correspondingly at the end-of-life stage (Corr et al., 2019). The four tasks refer to the physical task that aims to satisfy the needs of the physical body and minimize physical distress; the psychological task that aims to maximize psychological security, autonomy, and richness in living; the social task that aims to sustain and enhance interpersonal attachment, interaction, and relationship; and the spiritual task that aims to address the issues of meaningfulness, connectedness, and transcendence.

Consistent with the person-centred approach, an individual's choice and preference should be prioritized, as each individual should be allowed to decide which tasks and sets of tasks are important to him or her (Corr et al., 2019). The limited lifespan may not allow completion of all the tasks; some forms of assessment are therefore needed to locate the most urgent and important tasks that meet individual needs (Corr et al., 2019).

Supportive Care Framework for Cancer Care

Supportive care is defined as care that enhances the coping of patients and their families during illness diagnosis, treatment, death, and bereavement (Gysels et al., 2004). *Supportive care needs* refer to the required action or resource that is deemed necessary, desirable, or useful to achieve optimal wellbeing (Sanson-Fisher et al., 2000). Fitch (2008) formulates a framework that target the specific needs of patients with cancer, referred to as the Supportive Care Framework for Cancer Care. It builds on the constructs of human needs, cognitive appraisal, and coping as a foundation to conceptualize how a patient experiences and copes with cancer. It has been a tool for healthcare professionals to conceptualize their specific needs and for program managers to design and evaluate services tailored to them. It theorizes that cancer illness affects the fulfillment of needs across multiple life domains (Fitch, 2008). Seven needs are identified:

1. *Physical need*—the physical comfort and freedom from pain, optimum nutrition, ability to carry out one's usual day-to-day functions
2. *Emotional need*—a sense of comfort, belonging, understanding, and reassurance in times of stress and upset
3. *Social need*—family relationships, community acceptance, and involvement in relationships
4. *Psychological need*—the ability to cope with the illness experience and its consequences, including the need for optimal personal control and the need to experience positive self-esteem

5. *Spiritual need*—the meaning and purpose in life to practise religious beliefs
6. *Informational need*—information to reduce confusion, anxiety, and fear; to inform the person's or family's decision-making; and to assist in skill acquisition
7. *Practical need*—direct assistance to accomplish a task or activity and thereby reduce the demands on the person

Conclusions

As we reflect on the profound truth that "there is an end of cure; there is no end of care," it becomes clear that our focus must remain on providing continuous care and compassion. All the models discussed consistently emphasize the four core domains—physical, psychological, social, and spiritual—as the foundations of holistic, person-centred care. The subsequent chapters will elaborate on the traditional psychological interventions and the unmet needs of patients, structuring them within these four domains to ensure alignment with this comprehensive and compassionate approach.

References

Asadi-Lari, M., Tamburini, M., & Gray, D. (2004). Patients' needs, satisfaction, and health related quality of life: Towards a comprehensive model. *Health and Quality of Life Outcomes*, *2*(1), 32.

Beng, K. S. (2004). The last hours and days of life: A biopsychosocial-spiritual model of care. *Asia Pacific Family Medicine*, *4*, 1–3.

Borrell-Carrió, F., Suchman, A. L., & Epstein, R. M. (2004). The biopsychosocial model 25 years later: Principles, practice, and scientific inquiry. *Annals of Family Medicine*, *2*(6), 576–582.

Butow, P., & Tattersall, M. (2005). Shared decision making in cancer care. *Clinical Psychologist*, *9*, 54–58.

Corr, C. A. (1992). A task-based approach to coping with dying. *Omega, Journal of Death and Dying*, *24*, 81–94.

Corr, C. A., Corr, D. M., & Doka, K. J. (2019). *Death & dying, life & living* (8th ed.). Cengage.

Department of Health. (2000). *The NHS cancer plan*. Department of Health.

Engel, G. L. (1978). The biopsychosocial model and the education of health professionals. *Annals of the New York Academy of Sciences*, *310*(1), 169–181. https://doi.org/10.1111/j.1749-6632.1978.tb22070.x

Engel, G. L. (2012). The need for a new medical model: A challenge for biomedicine. *Psychodynamic Psychiatry*, *40*(3), 377–396. https://doi.org/10.1521/pdps.2012.40.3.377

Epstein, R., & Street, R. (2007). *Patient-centred communication in cancer care: Promoting healing and reducing suffering*. National Cancer Institute, NIH Publication.

Fitch, M. I. (2008). Supportive care framework. *The Canadian Oncology Nursing Journal*, *18*(1), 6–14.

Gysels, M., Higginson, I. J., Rajasekaran, M., Davies, E., & Harding, R. (2004). *Improving supportive and palliative care for adults with cancer: Research evidence.* National Institute of Clinical Excellence & Kings College London.

Institute of Medicine. (2001). *Crossing the quality chasm: A new health system for the 21st century.* National Academy Press.

Katerndahl, D. A. (2008). Impact of spiritual symptoms and their interactions on health services and life satisfaction. *Annals of Family Medicine, 6*(5), 412–420. https://doi.org/10.1370/afm.886

Mead, N., & Bower, P. (2000). Patient-centredness: A conceptual framework and review of the empirical literature. *Social Science & Medicine (1982), 51*(7), 1087–1110.

Sanson-Fisher, R., Girgis, A., Boyes, A., Bonevski, B., Burton, L., & Cook, P. (2000). The unmet supportive care needs of patients with cancer. Supportive care review group. *Cancer, 88*(1), 226–237.

Stewart, M. A. (1995). Effective physician-patient communication and health outcomes: A review. *CMAJ: Canadian Medical Association Journal = Journal de l'Association medicale canadienne, 152*(9), 1423–1433.

Sulmasy, D. (2002). A biopsychosocial-spiritual model for the care of patients at the end of life. *The Gerontologist, 42*(Suppl. 3), 24–33.

Verma, M. (2018). Magic word "palliative:" An end to cure but no end to care. *Indian Journal of Palliative Care, 24*(4), 545–546. https://doi.org/10.4103/IJPC.IJPC_86_18

World Health Organization. (2023). *Palliative care.* https://www.who.int/europe/news-room/fact-sheets/item/palliative-care

2 Traditional Psychological Interventions in Palliative Care

Introduction

"I am dying, how can you help me?"

At the heart of palliative care lies a profound understanding of the multifaceted needs of patients facing end-of-life challenges. With increasing scientific support, it becomes increasingly clear that psychological interventions play a crucial role in enhancing biopsychosocial spiritual care, offering relief without the side effects often associated with pharmaceutical treatments. This chapter begins by introducing the evidence-based psychological interventions traditionally practised in palliative care settings. These psychological interventions include cognitive behavioural therapy, mindfulness-based interventions, social support interventions, meaning-based interventions, and reminiscence and dignity therapy. After introducing the interventions with case studies, this chapter ends with a discussion of their limitations, with the next chapter discussing the unmet needs despite traditional pharmaceutical and psychological interventions. These discussions pave the way for the novel application of VR technology to intervene by providing special and immersive experiences.

Cognitive-behavioural Based Therapy

"Every time I struggle to breathe, it's a sign that I will die in the next second."

Cognitive behavioural therapy (CBT) has been a widely adopted approach in the field of palliative care, offering structured and effective interventions for symptom management. CBT is originally developed as a short-term and present-focused psychotherapy for the treatment of depression, while later to various mental disorders such as anxiety disorders and insomnia. Its core components include psychoeducation, cognitive reconstruction, relaxation, and exposure therapy. It emphasizes the intertwined relationship between

DOI: 10.4324/9781003518327-4

thoughts, emotions, behaviours, and physical sensations. It aims to identify and modify negative thinking patterns and beliefs that result in emotional distress and maladaptive behaviours (Alford & Beck, 1997; Beck, 2021; Serfaty et al., 2016). CBT is often used in palliative care settings to help patients cope with the psychological and emotional challenges associated with their symptoms, terminal illness, and existential challenges.

Benefits of CBT in Palliative Care

CBT has been found effective in managing the physical symptoms of patients with advanced diseases (Teo et al., 2019). Research results support the positive impact of CBT on reducing fatigue by modifying fatigue-related cognitions and behaviours (Abrahams et al., 2017; Poort et al., 2017). Psychoeducation delivered for end-stage renal disease has been found to improve symptoms and reduce acute hospital admissions (Chan et al., 2020), while those for patients with breast cancer reduce mood symptoms and uncertainty (Sato et al., 2023). Abundant studies have consistently demonstrated the efficacy of relaxation techniques for managing cancer-related symptoms (Dikmen & Terzioglu, 2019; Matsuda et al., 2014; Stoerkel et al., 2018).

In addition, CBT facilitates mood management in patients with advanced cancers (Azizoddin et al., 2024; Landa-Ramírez et al., 2020; Okuyama et al., 2017; Rayner et al., 2011; Traeger et al., 2012; Xia et al., 2024). Fulton et al. (2018) compare the efficacy of CBT with dignity-based interventions in reducing emotional symptoms and conclude that CBT is more efficacious, with a large effect size in reducing depressive symptoms and a small effect size in alleviating anxiety symptoms. The study also shows that interventions with more treatment sessions result in more significant reductions in depression symptoms. However, longer treatment sessions are associated with decreased improvement. The findings align with prior research (Anderson et al., 2008; Savard et al., 2006) suggesting that shorter sessions could be more appropriate for patients under palliative care, who may struggle with prolonged sessions due to their limited tolerance.

Case Study[1]

Mr. Alpha, a 68-year-old man diagnosed with stage IV lung cancer, currently stays at a residential care home for older adults. His primary concern is shortness of breath, which significantly impacts his quality of life. The difficulty in breathing not only causes physical discomfort but also leads to his fear that he is losing his breath. He also expresses feelings of inadequacy and helplessness in coping with the breathing difficulty. He expressed his wish to travel in natural environments, such as beaches and mountains, for a more peaceful mind.

How CBT can help Mr. Alpha

Psychoeducation. Psychoeducation on the relationship between Mr. Alpha's thoughts, behaviour, emotions, and physical sensations can help manage his symptoms of shortness of breath. It helps him gain insight into the impact of his thinking patterns on his emotional state and recognize the possible vicious cycle that perpetuates anxiety and shortness of breath. For instance, his anxious thought—Every time I struggle to breathe, it is a sign that I will die in the next second—can trigger anxiety and physiological responses, such as increased muscle tension and shallow breathing, which in turn exacerbate his physical symptoms and anxious thinking. With this knowledge, Mr. Alpha can proceed to learn cognitive strategies to reappraise his anxious thoughts, which helps reduce his anxiety level.

Cognitive interventions. Cognitive interventions assist Mr. Alpha in recognizing and evaluating his maladaptive thoughts related to his shortness of breath. The identified thought, "Every time I struggle to breathe, it is a sign that I will die in the next second," reflects his catastrophic cognition with the worst-case assumption that each episode of breathing difficulty impels immediate life threat. This thought aggravates his anxiety, which in turn intensifies his breathing difficulties. To address such maladaptive thoughts, the therapist can first help Mr. Alpha explore the evidence supporting and contradicting this thought. They can discuss past experiences when he encountered breathing difficulty but did not face life-threatening consequences. The therapist can explore with him the thinking errors that contribute to his catastrophic thinking. For example, the maladaptive thinking error "fortune-telling" that he assumes to know the future outcome without supportive evidence. The therapist can then help him generate alternative explanations for his difficulty breathing, such as the physical effects of his lung cancer or the presence of anxiety. Cognitive restructuring can be conducted to replace his catastrophic thoughts with more adaptive ones, such as "Although struggling to breathe is distressing, it does not necessarily mean that I will die in the next second. I have experienced this before and have managed to cope."

Behavioural interventions. Behavioural interventions can help Mr. Alpha manage his anxiety and shortness of breath. For instance, the therapist may coach deep breathing exercises to help him regulate his breathing. Through regular breathing practice, Mr. Alpha may develop a sense of control over his breathing difficulties. Mr. Alpha can be encouraged to engage in positive activities that bring him pleasure, calmness, and satisfaction. The therapist can explore activities with Mr. Alpha that align with his values and are within his physical capabilities. In light of his interest in nature, activities may include listening to music or watching videos with natural scenes.

Mindfulness-based Interventions

"I can't stop worrying! I want to get rid of my thinking!"

Mindfulness-based interventions have gained increasing recognition in palliative care in the past decade. It derives from the ancient Buddhist wisdom with growing support from modern psychological research. Mindfulness refers to "the awareness that emerges through paying attention on purpose, in the present moment, and nonjudgementally to the unfolding of experience moment by moment" (Kabat-Zinn, 2003). It is a practice that involves directing one's attention to the here and now, cultivating acceptance of the current experience, and fostering self-compassion. Standard mindfulness practices include meditation, focused breathing, and body scan exercises. With this awareness at the moment, individuals can develop a more accepting and non-judgemental relationship with their internal experiences, leading to positive psychological outcomes, such as reduced depression and anxiety (Hofmann & Gómez, 2017).

Benefits of Mindfulness in Palliative Care

Mindfulness plays an important role, particularly when patients struggle with incurable diseases. With the here-and-now focus, individuals may find peace in living each day to the fullest (von Blanckenburg & Leppin, 2018). Mindfulness-based interventions have shown moderate effects in reducing depression, anxiety, and cancer-specific distress while also promoting self-compassion and enhancing overall quality of life (Zimmermann et al., 2018). Mindful practices such as yoga and meditation have demonstrated positive effects on managing physical symptoms, including pain reduction in metastatic breast cancer patients (Carson et al., 2021).

Case Study

Mrs. Beta, a 72-year-old woman diagnosed with advanced breast cancer, currently stays at a residential care home for older adults. She presents with significant anxiety related to her illness. As a mother, she feels inadequate and sad about being unable to attend her daughter's upcoming wedding. She feels defeated every time when she tries to get rid of her worrying thoughts.

How Mindfulness-Based Interventions Can Help Mrs. Beta

Managing anxiety through present-moment awareness. Mrs. Beta can benefit from practising present-moment awareness through mindfulness techniques. She can be guided to observe her anxious thoughts without judgement and develop a sense of awareness. This aims to shift his attention from future-oriented thoughts to the present moment, thereby reducing anxiety related to her upcoming discharge and attendance at her daughter's wedding. She can learn and practise mindfulness techniques, such as mindful breathing exercises and body scans to observe sensations in her body, ultimately entering a relaxation state.

Facilitating acceptance of uncertainty. Mindfulness practice acknowledges the uncertainty of life and one's need for control. The therapist can help Mrs. Beta explore the acceptance towards the unpredictability of life and the truth that she cannot control every outcome. Instead, she can be helped to focus on what she can control in the present moment for a sense of calmness or self-compassion. She can also learn to treat herself with kindness and understanding with the realization that her worries and concerns are normal and natural.

Social Support Interventions

"I wish to go back home and have a dinner with my husband and children."

Social and emotional support is particularly essential for patients facing terminal illnesses (Bradley et al., 2018). It can enhance social connections, reduce loneliness, and provide a sense of belonging. It is recognized as an essential component of psychological interventions in palliative care (García-Rueda et al., 2016). Social support interventions should be tailored to the unique needs of individual patients to foster meaningful connections and a sense of companionship. In palliative care settings, social support may be limited by restrictions due to physical limitations, inadequate understanding from family and friends, and the impact of illness stigma on patients' relationships (Lloyd et al., 2016; Wilson & Luker, 2006; García-Rueda et al., 2016).

Benefits of Social Support Interventions in Palliative Care

Palliative care offers various interventions to facilitate social support and adaptive coping. These interventions include home visits, telecare services, activity groups, formal support groups, informal social activities, and the creation of dedicated environments such as palliative daycare centres (Bradley et al., 2022; Goodwin et al., 2002). Research has demonstrated the benefits of social support interventions in palliative care settings (Bradley et al.,

2011, 2018; Rush et al., 2023), which serve as protective factors against distress in patients with advanced cancer (Applebaum et al., 2014; Tomaka et al., 2006). Such social support has been linked to enhanced quality of life and reduced symptoms of depression and anxiety among patients with advanced cancer (Nipp et al., 2016). It has been found to help patients establish a sense of normality amidst their difficult circumstances (Lobb et al., 2015). In a study conducted by Steineck et al. (2021), adolescents and young adults with advanced cancer cite digital technologies as a helpful platform for maintaining peer relationships and seeking psychosocial support, unveiling the potential of digital support interventions.

Case Study

Mrs. Charlie, a 68-year-old woman with advanced pancreatic cancer, now stays in an isolated room of a residential unit for older adults for infection control. Given the restricted visiting hours, she feels lonely and disconnected from her usual social support networks. She longs for companionship and emotional support. She wishes to reunite with her husband and have a heartfelt dinner with children at her own home.

How Social Support Interventions Can Help Mrs. Charlie

Visits from friends, family members, or healthcare professionals, such as social workers or counselors, can offer comfort, reassurance, and understanding to Mrs. Charlie. These companions can engage in meaningful activities with her, such as engaging her in conversations or providing a sense of companionship. If face-to-face contact is not allowed for infection control, video calls or social media platforms can be used to enable virtual visits with loved ones.

Meaning-Based Interventions

"What's the point of staying alive?!"

Inspired by existential philosophy and derived from the profound experiences of the world wars, meaning-based interventions acknowledge that individuals can create meaning in their lives even in the face of adversity. These interventions focus on helping individuals explore personal values, connect life with a sense of purpose, and foster a sense of legacy and continuity. Particularly in the face of terminal illnesses, individuals may encounter existential distress, such as death anxiety, loss of roles, feelings of isolation, and regrets (Breitbart et al., 2018). Meaning-based interventions address these challenges by exploring existential themes and searching for meaning. These interventions aim to help patients cope with loss, redefine life goals, and reevaluate missed opportunities (Guerrero-Torrelles et al., 2017).

Benefits of Meaning-based Interventions in Palliative Care

Meaning-centred psychotherapy (MCP) refers to therapeutic approaches designed to enhance meaning, spiritual well-being, and quality of life (Thomas et al., 2014). It has shown promise in the therapeutic benefits among patients with advanced cancers (Kang et al., 2019; Lethborg et al., 2019; Rodin & Hales, 2021; Teo et al., 2019). Results of a large randomized controlled trial show that individual MCP significantly improves overall quality of life, sense of meaning, and spiritual well-being compared to supportive therapy and enhanced usual care (Rosenfeld et al., 2018; Breitbart et al., 2018). One example is Managing Cancer and Living Meaningfully (CALM) intervention which is specifically designed for advanced cancer patients. CALM intervention is reported to reduce symptoms of depression compared to those receiving treatment as usual (Rodin et al., 2018). CALM interventions provide structured sessions focusing on symptom management, communication with healthcare professionals, finding meaning and purpose, self-transformation, relationship dynamics, and addressing concerns about the future and death. A study by Wagner et al. (2016) reports the feasibility and efficacy of meaning-based intervention for patients with advanced cancer and their spouses.

Case Study

Mrs. Delta, a 78-year-old woman, is currently facing the challenges of metastatic cancer and cord compression. These conditions have left her bedbound, requiring specialized care in a rehabilitation hospital. She presents with unresolved pain and emotional distress. When adjusting to tetraplegia, she expresses a sense of meaninglessness and a passive death wish. Mrs. Delta feels frustrated and saddened by her physical limitations, which have impacted her ability to engage in activities she once enjoyed. She is concerned about her ability to fulfill her mother's role and struggles with feelings of worthlessness. She also expressed her wish to see the aurora borealis, which has been the dream of her life.

How Meaning-Based Interventions Can Help Mrs. Delta

Clarifying personal values and goals. Meaning-based interventions can help Mrs. Delta identify her core values and what is truly important to her. She might be guided in reflecting on her fondest memories or cherished relationships. She might be helped to acknowledge her own competence and effort in raising her children and her unfailing support to her beloved family. Through clarifying her values, Mrs. Delta can make decisions and take actions that align with her priorities, for example, initiating open and meaningful conversations with her husband and children to deepen the emotional bond and enhance their understanding of her perspective. They may reminisce about shared memories, express gratitude and love, and talk about her last wishes of viewing the aurora borealis.

Exploring meaning and purpose. The therapist can help Mrs. Delta explore her resilience and strengths in the face of her physical limitations. Exercise may help highlight moments of resilience and triumph throughout her life, reminding her of her adaptive coping. Through the acknowledgement, Mrs. Delta can find encouragement for herself and become a role model for her children, inspiring them to face their own difficulties with determination and resilience. The therapist can also help Mrs. Delta reflect on her life experiences and identify the wisdom she wishes to pass on to her children and future generations. She may engage in activities such as recording audio messages or creating a memory book with the therapist's assistance.

Reminiscence and Dignity Therapy

"Do you mind listening to my stories?"

Reminiscence and dignity therapy refers to the process of recalling past experiences, allowing individuals to reflect on unresolved conflicts and reintegrate their life experiences. It aims to improve self-esteem and foster a sense of fulfillment by assisting individuals in reviewing their past experiences (Butler, 1963; O'Philbin et al., 2018; Park et al., 2019). This therapy uses prompts or cues such as photos, videos, music, or objects. Through reviewing life events, individuals can work towards resolving the developmental stage of ego integrity versus despair, which is proposed by psychosocial theory (Erikson, 1950). Dignity therapy is similar to reminiscence therapy but emphasizes creating a legacy document that captures significant past events in a patient's life (Vuksanovic et al., 2016). Such legacy documents may bring therapeutic benefits, allowing individuals to leave behind memories, values, or messages for their loved ones.

Benefits of Reminiscence and Dignity Therapy in Palliative Care

Reminiscence therapy has been found to enhance communication and alleviate psychological and behavioural symptoms such as depression and agitation (O'Philbin et al., 2018; Park et al., 2019), while dignity therapy has shown positive effects on existential distress, addressing the emotional and psychological needs of patients (Julião et al., 2017). Systematic reviews focusing on these two interventions in patients with advanced cancer have reported their therapeutic benefits in spiritual well-being and overall quality of life (Martínez et al., 2017; Wang et al., 2017). Involving the patient's family or significant others in the therapy process has been associated with reduced feelings of isolation and despair, as well as improved communication and connectedness (Guo et al., 2018; Ho et al., 2017). Systematic reviews conclude with promising evidence of life review interventions among patients with advanced cancers (Teo et al., 2019; Wang et al., 2017).

Case Study

Mrs. Echo is an 85-year-old woman with end-stage renal disease. She is bored at hostel and eager to share her personal views and experiences. Her illness and the resulting physical restrictions have limited her activities, leading to a sense of purposelessness in her daily life. Mrs. Echo yearns to connect with others and share about her life experiences.

How Reminiscence Therapy Can Help Mrs. Echo

Life review and meaning-making. Reminiscence therapy allows Mrs. Echo to engage in a life review process, which reflects on the significant life events, decisions, and lessons learned. A life storybook or diagram can be created that documents significant events, milestones, and memories from her life. She can be guided to reflect on and integrate her life story to facilitate a sense of agency over her narrative. This life storybook or diagram can be shared with loved ones, which allows others to have a deeper understanding of Mrs. Echo's life and experiences. Throughout the process, her life experiences are validated with her needs and values listened to.

Limitations of Traditional Psychological Interventions

"I feel better after our conversations, but I still want to escape from my isolation room and immerse myself in the mountains."

Despite the therapeutic benefits of traditional psychological interventions, the traditional approaches elaborated in this chapter have their limitations and specific challenges that warrant innovative approaches that help make up for the shortcomings. For CBT, accessibility to professional services has been a significant challenge, leading to the exploration of cost-effective alternatives such as digital interventions (Cheung et al., 2017). Mindfulness-based interventions require adaptations to overcome barriers such as treatment duration (Zimmermann et al., 2018). Social support interventions call for innovative and technological approaches when considering the high prevalence of limited physical mobility in the palliative care population (Owen et al., 2017). Meaning-based interventions require a person-centred approach, allowing patients to guide the treatment focus based on their own preferences (Rosenfeld et al., 2017). Reminiscence and dignity therapy relies heavily on the expertise of the therapists (Liu et al., 2021; Yue & Chen, 2013), with gerontological social workers or psychologists recommended for optimal outcomes (Chiang et al., 2010).

Even with the implementation of traditional interventions, a number of patients' clinical needs are unresolved, as revealed by the five case studies discussed in this chapter. Mr. Alpha, who underwent CBT, still longs to travel and immerse himself in nature despite the cognitive and behavioural interventions. Mrs. Beta's unmet emotional needs persist as she cannot participate in the upcoming wedding of her beloved daughter. Mrs. Charlie still feels sad being unable to return home and have dinner with her family. Despite meaning-based interventions, Mrs. Delta cannot manage to enjoy the aurora borealis to complete her bucket list. Mrs. Echo's engagement in stimulating activities within the hostel setting is still limited, even with traditional reminiscence therapy.

Conclusions

In the compassionate landscape of palliative care, traditional psychological interventions have long been essential in addressing the biopsychosocial-spiritual needs of patients facing life-limiting illnesses. However, despite their importance, these interventions often fall short, leaving some clinical needs unmet. These unmet needs, which will be further elaborated on in the next chapter, highlight the necessity for innovative interventions, such as the use of VR technology to address the previously mentioned challenges and provide new avenues for fulfillment and well-being. The case studies elaborated in this chapter will be further examined in Section III to demonstrate how VR technology can complement traditional psychological interventions through its immersive and tailored experience.

Note

1 Please note that the case study presented throughout the book is a hypothetical scenario and does not contain real patient information.

References

Abrahams, H. J. G., Gielissen, M. F. M., Donders, R. R. T., Goedendorp, M. M., van der Wouw, A. J., Verhagen, C. A. H. H. V. M., & Knoop, H. (2017). The efficacy of internet-based cognitive behavioral therapy for severely fatigued survivors of breast cancer compared with care as usual: A randomized controlled trial. *Cancer*, *123*(19), 3825–3834. https://doi.org/10.1002/cncr.30815

Alford, B. A., & Beck, A. T. (1997). *The integrative power of cognitive therapy*. Guilford Press.

Anderson, T., Watson, M., & Davidson, R. (2008). The use of cognitive behavioural therapy techniques for anxiety and depression in hospice patients: A feasibility study. *Palliative Medicine*, *22*(7), 814–821. https://doi.org/10.1177/0269216308095157

Applebaum, A. J., Stein, E. M., Lord-Bessen, J., Pessin, H., Rosenfeld, B., & Breitbart, W. (2014). Optimism, social support, and mental health outcomes in patients with advanced cancer: Optimism, social support, and advanced cancer. *Psycho-Oncology (Chichester, England)*, *23*(3), 299–306. https://doi.org/10.1002/pon.3418

Azizoddin, D. R., DeForge, S. M., Baltazar, A., Edwards, R. R., Allsop, M., Tulsky, J. A., Businelle, M. S., Schreiber, K. L., & Enzinger, A. C. (2024). Development and pre-pilot testing of STAMP + CBT: An mHealth app combining pain cognitive behavioral therapy and opioid support for patients with advanced cancer and pain. *Supportive Care in Cancer*, *32*(2), 123. https://doi.org/10.1007/s00520-024-08307-7

Beck, J. S. (2021). *Cognitive behavior therapy: Basics and beyond* (3rd ed.). The Guilford Press.

Bradley, N. M., Dowrick, C. F., & Lloyd-Williams, M. (2022). A survey of hospice day services in the United Kingdom & Republic of Ireland: How did hospices offer social support to palliative care patients, pre-pandemic? *BMC Palliative Care*, *21*(1), 1–170. https://doi.org/10.1186/s12904-022-01061-9

Bradley, N. M., Lloyd-Williams, M., & Dowrick, C. (2018). Effectiveness of palliative care interventions offering social support to people with life-limiting illness—a systematic review. *European Journal of Cancer Care*, *27*(3), e12837. https://doi.org/10.1111/ecc.12837

Bradley, S. E., Frizelle, D., & Johnson, M. (2011). Patients' psychosocial experiences of attending specialist palliative day care: A systematic review. *Palliative Medicine*, *25*(3), 210–228. https://doi.org/10.1177/0269216310389222

Breitbart, W., Pessin, H., Rosenfeld, B., Applebaum, A. J., Lichtenthal, W. G., Li, Y., Saracino, R. M., Marziliano, A. M., Masterson, M., Tobias, K., & Fenn, N. (2018). Individual meaning-centered psychotherapy for the treatment of psychological and existential distress: A randomized controlled trial in patients with advanced cancer. *Cancer*, *124*(15), 3231–3239. https://doi.org/10.1002/cncr.31539

Butler, R. N. (1963). The life review: An interpretation of reminiscence in the aged. *Psychiatry*, *26*, 65–76. https://doi.org/10.1080/00332747.1963.11023339

Carson, J. W., Carson, K. M., Olsen, M., Sanders, L., Westbrook, K., Keefe, F. J., & Porter, L. S. (2021). Yoga practice predicts improvements in day-to-day pain in women with metastatic breast cancer. *Journal of Pain and Symptom Management*, *61*(6), 1227–1233. https://doi.org/10.1016/j.jpainsymman.2020.10.009

Chan, K.-Y., Yip, T., Yap, D. Y. H., Sham, M. K., & Tsang, K. W. (2020). A pilot comprehensive psychoeducation program for fluid management in renal palliative care patients: Impact on health care utilization. *Journal of Palliative Medicine*, *23*(11), 1518–1524. https://doi.org/10.1089/jpm.2019.0424

Charalambous, A., Giannakopoulou, M., Bozas, E., Marcou, Y., Kitsios, P., & Paikousis, L. (2016). Guided imagery and progressive muscle relaxation as a cluster of symptoms management intervention in patients receiving chemotherapy: A randomized control trial. *PloS One, 11*(6), e0156911.

Cheung, E. O., Cohn, M. A., Dunn, L. B., Melisko, M. E., Morgan, S., Penedo, F. J., Salsman, J. M., Shumay, D. M., & Moskowitz, J. T. (2017). A randomized pilot trial of a positive affect skill intervention (lessons in linking affect and coping) for women with metastatic breast cancer. *Psycho-Oncology (Chichester, England), 26*(12), 2101–2108. https://doi.org/10.1002/pon.4312

Chiang, K. J., Chu, H., Chang, H. J., Chung, M. H., Chen, C. H., Chiou, H. Y., & Chou, K. R. (2010). The effects of reminiscence therapy on psychological well-being, depression, and loneliness among the institutionalized aged. *International Journal of Geriatric Psychiatry, 25*(4), 380–388. https://doi.org/10.1002/gps.2350

Dikmen, H. A., & Terzioglu, F. (2019). Effects of reflexology and progressive muscle relaxation on pain, fatigue, and quality of life during chemotherapy in gynecologic cancer patients. *Pain Management Nursing, 20*(1), 47–53.

Erikson, E. H. (1950). *Childhood and society.* W. W. Norton & Co.

Fulton, J. J., Newins, A. R., Porter, L. S., & Ramos, K. (2018). Psychotherapy targeting depression and anxiety for use in palliative care: A meta-analysis. *Journal of Palliative Medicine, 21*(7), 124–1037. https://doi.org/10.1089/jpm.2017.0576

García-Rueda, N., Carvajal Valcárcel, A., Saracíbar-Razquin, M., & Arantzamendi Solabarrieta, M. (2016). The experience of living with advanced-stage cancer: A thematic synthesis of the literature. *European Journal of Cancer Care, 25*(4), 551–569. https://doi.org/10.1111/ecc.12523

Goodwin, D. M., Higginson, I. J., Myers, K., Douglas, H. R., & Normand, C. E. (2002). What is palliative day care? A patient perspective of five UK services. *Supportive Care in Cancer, 10*(7), 556–562. https://doi.org/10.1007/s00520-002-0380-1

Guerrero-Torrelles, M., Monforte-Royo, C., Rodríguez-Prat, A., Porta-Sales, J., & Balaguer, A. (2017). Understanding meaning in life interventions in patients with advanced disease: A systematic review and realist synthesis. *Palliative Medicine, 31*(9), 798–813. https://doi.org/10.1177/0269216316685235

Guo, Q., Chochinov, H. M., McClement, S., Thompson, G., & Hack, T. (2018). Development and evaluation of the dignity talk question framework for palliative patients and their families: A mixed-methods study. *Palliative Medicine, 32*(1), 195–205. https://doi.org/10.1177/0269216317734696

Ho, A. H. Y., Car, J., Ho, M.-H. R., Tan-Ho, G., Choo, P. Y., Patinadan, P. V., Chong, P. H., Ong, W. Y., Fan, G., Tan, Y. P., Neimeyer, R. A., & Chochinov, H. M. (2017). A novel family dignity intervention (FDI) for enhancing and informing holistic palliative care in Asia: Study protocol for a randomized controlled trial. *Current Controlled Trials in Cardiovascular Medicine, 18*(1), 587. https://doi.org/10.1186/s13063-017-2325-5

Hofmann, S. G., & Gómez, A. F. (2017). Mindfulness-based interventions for anxiety and depression. *The Psychiatric Clinics of North America, 40*(4), 739–749. https://doi.org/10.1016/j.psc.2017.08.008

Julião, M., Oliveira, F., Nunes, B., Carneiro, A. V., & Barbosa, A. (2017). Effect of dignity therapy on end-of-life psychological distress in terminally ill Portuguese patients: A randomized controlled trial. *Palliative & Supportive Care, 15*(6), 628–637. https://doi.org/10.1017/S1478951516001140

Kabat-Zinn, J. (2003). Mindfulness-based interventions in context: Past, present, and future. *Clinical Psychology (New York, N.Y.), 10*(2), 144–156. https://doi.org/10.1093/clipsy.bpg016

Kang, K.-A., Han, S.-J., Lim, Y.-S., & Kim, S.-J. (2019). Meaning-centered interventions for patients with advanced or terminal cancer: A meta-analysis. *Cancer Nursing, 42*(4), 332–340. https://doi.org/10.1097/NCC.0000000000000628

Landa-Ramírez, E., Greer, J. A., Sánchez-Román, S., Manolov, R., Salado-Avila, M. M., Templos-Esteban, L. A., & Riveros-Rosas, A. (2020). Tailoring cognitive behavioral therapy for depression and anxiety symptoms in Mexican terminal cancer patients: A multiple baseline study. *Journal of Clinical Psychology in Medical Settings*, *27*(1), 54–67. https://doi.org/10.1007/s10880-019-09620-8

Lethborg, C., Kissane, D. W., & Schofield, P. (2019). Meaning and purpose (MaP) therapy I: Therapeutic processes and themes in advanced cancer. *Palliative & Supportive Care*, *17*(1), 13–20. https://doi.org/10.1017/S1478951518000871

Liu, Z., Yang, F., Lou, Y., Zhou, W., & Tong, F. (2021). The effectiveness of reminiscence therapy on alleviating depressive symptoms in older adults: A systematic review. *Frontiers in Psychology*, *12*, 709853. https://doi.org/10.3389/fpsyg.2021.709853

Lloyd, A., Kendall, M., Starr, J. M., & Murray, S. A. (2016). Physical, social, psychological and existential trajectories of loss and adaptation towards the end of life for older people living with frailty: A serial interview study. *BMC Geriatrics*, *16*(1), 176. https://doi.org/10.1186/s12877-016-0350-y

Lobb, E. A., Lacey, J., Kearsley, J., Liauw, W., White, L., & Hosie, A. (2015). Living with advanced cancer and an uncertain disease trajectory: An emerging patient population in palliative care? *BMJ Supportive & Palliative Care*, *5*(4), 352–357. https://doi.org/10.1136/bmjspcare-2012-000381

Martínez, M., Arantzamendi, M., Belar, A., Carrasco, J. M., Carvajal, A., Rullán, M., & Centeno, C. (2017). 'Dignity therapy', a promising intervention in palliative care: A comprehensive systematic literature review. *Palliative medicine*, *31*(6), 492–509. https://doi.org/10.1177/0269216316665562

Matsuda, A., Yamaoka, K., Tango, T., Matsuda, T., & Nishimoto, H. (2014). Effectiveness of psychoeducational support on quality of life in early-stage breast cancer patients: A systematic review and meta-analysis of randomized controlled trials. *Quality of Life Research*, *23*, 21–30.

Nipp, R. D., El-Jawahri, A., Fishbein, J. N., Eusebio, J., Stagl, J. M., Gallagher, E. R., Park, E. R., Jackson, V. A., Pirl, W. F., Greer, J. A., & Temel, J. S. (2016). The relationship between coping strategies, quality of life, and mood in patients with incurable cancer. *Cancer*, *122*(13), 2110–2116. https://doi.org/10.1002/cncr.30025

Okuyama, T., Akechi, T., Mackenzie, L., & Furukawa, T. A. (2017). Psychotherapy for depression among advanced, incurable cancer patients: A systematic review and meta-analysis. *Cancer Treatment Reviews*, *56*, 16–27. https://doi.org/10.1016/j.ctrv.2017.03.012

O'Philbin, L., Woods, B., Farrell, E. M., Spector, A. E., & Orrell, M. (2018). Reminiscence therapy for dementia: An abridged Cochrane systematic review of the evidence from randomized controlled trials. *Expert Review of Neurotherapeutics*, *18*(9), 715–727.

Owen, J. E., O'Carroll Bantum, E., Pagano, I. S., & Stanton, A. (2017). Randomized trial of a social networking intervention for cancer-related distress. *Annals of Behavioral Medicine*, *51*(5), 661–672. https://doi.org/10.1007/s12160-017-9890-4

Park, K., Lee, S., Yang, J., Song, T., & Hong, G.-R. S. (2019). A systematic review and meta-analysis on the effect of reminiscence therapy for people with dementia. *International Psychogeriatrics*, *31*(11), 1581–1597.

Poort, H., Verhagen, C. A. H. H. V. M., Peters, M. E. W. J., Goedendorp, M. M., Donders, A. R. T., Hopman, M. T. E., Nijhuis-van der Sanden, M. W. G., Berends, T., Bleijenberg, G., & Knoop, H. (2017). Study protocol of the TIRED study:

A randomised controlled trial comparing either graded exercise therapy for severe fatigue or cognitive behaviour therapy with usual care in patients with incurable cancer. *BMC Cancer, 17*(1), 81. https://doi.org/10.1186/s12885-017-3076-0

Rayner, L., Price, A., Hotopf, M., & Higginson, I. J. (2011). The development of evidence-based European guidelines on the management of depression in palliative cancer care. *European Journal of Cancer (Oxford, England: 1990), 47*(5), 702–712. https://doi.org/10.1016/j.ejca.2010.11.027

Rodin, G., & Hales, S. A. (2021). *Managing cancer and living meaningfully: An evidence-based intervention for cancer patients and their caregivers.* Oxford University Press.

Rodin, G., Lo, C., Rydall, A., Shnall, J., Malfitano, C., Chiu, A., Panday, T., Watt, S., An, E., Nissim, R., Li, M., Zimmermann, C., & Hales, S. (2018). Managing cancer and living meaningfully (CALM): A randomized controlled trial of a psychological intervention for patients with advanced cancer. *Journal of Clinical Oncology, 36*(23), 2422–2432. https://doi.org/10.1200/JCO.2017.77.1097

Rosenfeld, B., Cham, H., Pessin, H., & Breitbart, W. (2018). Why is meaning-centered group psychotherapy (MCGP) effective? Enhanced sense of meaning as the mechanism of change for advanced cancer patients. *Psycho-Oncology (Chichester, England), 27*(2), 654–660. https://doi.org/10.1002/pon.4578

Rosenfeld, B., Saracino, R., Tobias, K., Masterson, M., Pessin, H., Applebaum, A., Brescia, R., & Breitbart, W. (2017). Adapting meaning-centered psychotherapy for the palliative care setting: Results of a pilot study. *Palliative Medicine, 31*(2), 140–146. https://doi.org/10.1177/0269216316651570

Rush, C. L., Lester, E. G., Berry, J. D., Brizzi, K. T., Lindenberger, E. C., Curtis, J. R., & Vranceanu, A.-M. (2023). A roadmap for early psychosocial support in palliative care for people impacted by ALS—reducing suffering, building resiliency, and setting the stage for delivering timely transdiagnostic psychosocial care. *Translational Behavioral Medicine, 13*(9), 722–726. https://doi.org/10.1093/tbm/ibad024

Sato, T., Seto, M., Sangai, T., Norihiko, S., Nishimiya, H., Kikuchi, M., Shimizu, A., & Iwamitsu, Y. (2023). The effectiveness of pretreatment video-based psychoeducation for patients with breast cancer. *Palliative & Supportive Care, 21*(6), 1016–1023. https://doi.org/10.1017/S1478951523001372

Savard, J., Simard, S., Giguère, I., Ivers, H., Morin, C. M., Maunsell, E., Gagnon, P., Robert, J., & Marceau, D. (2006). Randomized clinical trial on cognitive therapy for depression in women with metastatic breast cancer: Psychological and immunological effects. *Palliative & Supportive Care, 4*(3), 219–237. https://doi.org/10.1017/S1478951506060305

Serfaty, M., King, M., Nazareth, I., Tookman, A., Wood, J., Gola, A., Aspden, T., Mannix, K., Davis, S., Moorey, S., & Jones, L. (2016). The clinical and cost effectiveness of cognitive behavioural therapy plus treatment as usual for the treatment of depression in advanced cancer (CanTalk): Study protocol for a randomised controlled trial. *Current Controlled Trials in Cardiovascular Medicine, 17*(1), 113. https://doi.org/10.1186/s13063-016-1223-6

Steineck, A., Walsh, C., Barton, K., Yi-Frazier, J., & Rosenberg, A. (2021). Seeking virtual support: Social media in the advanced cancer experience among adolescents and young adults (AYAs) (SCI941). *Journal of Pain and Symptom Management, 61*(3), 691–692. https://doi.org/10.1016/j.jpainsymman.2021.01.102

Stoerkel, E., Bellanti, D., Paat, C., Peacock, K., Aden, J., Setlik, R., Walter, J., & Inman, A. (2018). Effectiveness of a self-care toolkit for surgical breast cancer patients in a military treatment facility. *The Journal of Alternative and Complementary Medicine, 24*(9–10), 916–925.

Teo, I., Krishnan, A., & Lee, G. L. (2019). Psychosocial interventions for advanced cancer patients: A systematic review. *Psycho-Oncology (Chichester, England)*, *28*(7), 1394–1407. https://doi.org/10.1002/pon.5103

Thomas, L. P., Meier, E. A., & Irwin, S. A. (2014). Meaning-centered psychotherapy: A form of psychotherapy for patients with cancer. *Current Psychiatry Reports*, *16*(10), 488. https://doi.org/10.1007/s11920-014-0488-2

Tomaka, J., Thompson, S., & Palacios, R. (2006). The relation of social isolation, loneliness, and social support to disease outcomes among the elderly. *Journal of Aging and Health*, *18*(3), 359–384. https://doi.org/10.1177/0898264305280993

Traeger, L., Greer, J. A., Fernandez-Robles, C., Temel, J. S., & Pirl, W. F. (2012). Evidence-based treatment of anxiety in patients with cancer. *Journal of Clinical Oncology*, *30*(11), 1197–1205. https://doi.org/10.1200/JCO.2011.39.5632

von Blanckenburg, P., & Leppin, N. (2018). Psychological interventions in palliative care. *Current Opinion in Psychiatry*, *31*(5), 389–395. https://doi.org/10.1097/YCO.0000000000000441

Vuksanovic, D., Green, H. J., Dyck, M., & Morrissey, S. A. (2016). Dignity therapy and life review for palliative care patients: A randomised controlled trial. *Journal of Pain and Symptom Management*, *53*(2), 162–170.e1. https://doi.org/10.1016/j.jpainsymman.2016.09.005

Wagner, C. D., Johns, S., Brown, L. F., Hanna, N., & Bigatti, S. M. (2016). Acceptability and feasibility of a meaning-based intervention for patients with advanced cancer and their spouses: A pilot study. *American Journal of Hospice & Palliative Medicine*, *33*(6), 546–554. https://doi.org/10.1177/1049909115575709

Wang, C. W., Chow, A. Y., & Chan, C. L. (2017). The effects of life review interventions on spiritual well-being, psychological distress, and quality of life in patients with terminal or advanced cancer: A systematic review and meta-analysis of randomized controlled trials. *Palliative Medicine*, *31*(10), 883–894. https://doi.org/10.1177/0269216317705101

Wilson, K., & Luker, K. A. (2006). At home in hospital? Interaction and stigma in people affected by cancer. *Social Science & Medicine (1982)*, *62*(7), 1616–1627. https://doi.org/10.1016/j.socscimed.2005.08.053

Xia, W., Zheng, Y., Guo, D., Zhu, Y., & Tian, L. (2024). Effects of cognitive behavioral therapy on anxiety and depressive symptoms in advanced cancer patients: A meta-analysis. *General Hospital Psychiatry*, *87*, 20–32. https://doi.org/10.1016/j.genhosppsych.2024.01.006

Yue, Y., & Chen, Y. Y. (2013). Effect of structured group reminiscence on depressive symptoms and life satisfaction in elders. *China Modern Doctor*, *51*, 110–112. [Google Scholar].

Zimmermann, F. F., Burrell, B., & Jordan, J. (2018). The acceptability and potential benefits of mindfulness-based interventions in improving psychological well-being for adults with advanced cancer: A systematic review. *Complementary Therapies in Clinical Practice*, *30*, 68–78. https://doi.org/10.1016/j.ctcp.2017.12.014

3 Unmet Needs in Palliative Care

Introduction

In the previous chapter, I introduced evidence-based psychological approaches that strive to enhance the quality of life for patients in palliative care. Despite the progress we have made, it is essential to acknowledge that many fundamental needs remain unmet by conventional psychological and pharmaceutical methods. This chapter takes a closer look at the unaddressed needs of patients at the end-of-life stage through the lens of the biopsychosocial–spiritual model. It also explores the unmet needs, such as inadequate advance care planning and support for palliative care providers. The chapter aims to shed light on the service gaps in palliative care, which allow innovative technologies, such as VR, to step in to address the unmet needs.

Unmet Physical Needs

"I'm still in pain, despite pain killers."

Pain

Unresolved pain is one of the prominent unmet needs. According to a systematic review conducted by Wang et al. (2018), 75% of patients under palliative care consider pain as an unmet need. Van den Beuken-van Everdingen et al. (2016) similarly report in another systematic review that more than one-third of patients experiencing moderate or severe pain and approximately two-thirds of patients with metastatic, terminal, or advanced illness reporting pain. Apart from the high prevalence and intensity of pain, patients under palliative care experience pain in multiple locations and with varying patterns (Wilkie & Ezenwa, 2012).

The use of analgesics is a common strategy for pain management. The World Health Organization (WHO) proposes the WHO analgesic ladder,

DOI: 10.4324/9781003518327-5

with the first step recommending that medical doctors treat patients using non-opioid analgesics. If the patient continues to experience pain, doctors are advised to step up to using mild opioids. If the pain still cannot be managed, doctors may proceed to the highest level and use strong opioids (Anekar et al., 2023). According to a systematic review by Azevedo São Leão Ferreira et al. (2006) on the effectiveness of the WHO analgesic ladder, when applied correctly, the advice offered by the ladder helps 45% to 100% of patients to adequately relieve pain.

Although the WHO analgesic ladder is helpful for some patients under palliative care, a portion of patients may encounter unresolved pain due to practical issues. Some types of pain, such as neuropathic pain, which is described by patients as a burning, aching, and penetrating kind of pain (Dobratz, 2009), do not respond well to the typical analgesics recommended by the WHO analgesic ladder. Neuropathic pain is caused by a lesion or illness that affects the nervous system (Leppert et al., 2016). Opioids, an analgesic suggested at the highest level of the WHO analgesic ladder, are ineffective for treating neuropathic pain, as such pain affects various regions of the central and peripheral nervous systems (Anekar et al., 2023).

In addition, some patient-related factors limit effective pain management. A systematic review by Jacobsen et al. (2009) reveals three patient-related obstacles to cancer pain management. First, patients may be reluctant to use analgesics due to concerns about addiction and tolerance, side effects, and newly-developed symptoms being concealed by analgesics. Second, patients may not communicate well with their medical doctors or report their pain accurately. They may perceive that talking about pain makes them a "bad patient," or believe that pain relief is not a primary concern for doctors. Third, patients may believe that pain is uncontrollable and/or that cancer-related pain is inevitable.

These patient-related obstacles negatively influence patient's pain experiences. Negative beliefs about analgesics can directly lead to high pain intensity despite adherence to the prescribed pain management regimen. Patients' negative beliefs also adversely impact their ability to communicate their pain effectively and/or adhere to the recommended treatment plan (Jacobsen et al., 2009). Although pharmacotherapy has been widely adopted for pain management, practical and patient-related obstacles exist that limit its effectiveness and render pain an unmet need for patients under palliative care.

Fatigue

Fatigue is another significant physical concern in end-of-life care. Fatigue refers to the subjective experience of lacking energy or general weakness (Radbruch et al., 2008). Patients experiencing fatigue often describe themselves as being like "a zombie," "a wet fish," or a "carpet," and completely drained of energy (Scott et al., 2011). A cross-sectional survey by Wang et al. (2021) reports that 69% of Chinese patients under palliative care are distressed by fatigue, while a systematic review by Wang et al. (2018) finds that up to 76% of patients with advanced cancer report fatigue as an unmet need.

Two kinds of fatigue are experienced by patients with terminal illnesses: peripheral fatigue and central fatigue. *Peripheral fatigue* refers to the inability of muscles to generate strength, whereas *central fatigue* refers to the failure to maintain sufficient control for driving muscle actions (Borneman, 2013). Yavuzsen et al. (2009) report that patients with cancer-related fatigue have higher levels of central fatigue than healthy individuals. As a result, patients under palliative care may find it challenging to use their muscles consistently to perform tasks that require continuous physical effort. Research has shown that the ongoing lack of energy leads to limited social and familial interactions for patients, as well as difficulties in thinking and feelings of anger or frustration (Scott et al., 2011), all of which ultimately impede the quality of patients' end-of-life.

Various interventions have been explored for the management of fatigue. Physical exercise has been extensively studied and has been found to provide consistent yet minor benefits (Fuller et al., 2018). Educational programmes that emphasize managing instead of treating fatigue have been delivered (Bennett et al., 2016), while psychological interventions aim to target distorted perceptions of fatigue or maladaptive coping strategies (Corbett et al., 2019). More robust research is needed on the effectiveness of complementary therapies, such as massage and acupuncture, and pharmacological treatments for managing fatigue in palliative care (Dean, 2019). Overall, there appears to be no one-size-fits-all approach for managing fatigue among patients in palliative care.

Similar to when experiencing pain, there are several reasons why patients in palliative care may be reluctant to report fatigue. They may think that fatigue is inevitable and untreatable, which may lead to a sense of hopelessness and the perception that interventions are not helpful (Shun et al., 2011; Stone et al., 2000). Some patients may worry that expressing fatigue may negatively affect their medical treatment, possibly reducing or terminating treatment (Berger et al., 2015; Shun et al., 2009), while some may fear that fatigue indicates a poor response to treatment or a worsening of their illness (Borneman, 2013). It appears that an effective method of managing fatigue has yet to be identified, leaving fatigue as one of the unresolved needs for palliative care patients.

Sleep Problems

Patients under palliative care often encounter sleep problems, such as difficulties initiating sleep, difficulties staying asleep, early morning awakening, or having a non-restorative sleep with low sleep efficiency (Savard & Morin, 2001). An observational study conducted by Mercadante et al. (2015) reports 24% to 95% of patients under palliative care having sleep-related issues, while a systematic review by Nzwalo et al. (2020) investigating insomnia among patients under palliative care highlights that at least one-third have sleep problems.

Spielman's three-factor model (Spielman et al., 1987) outlines the factors that may contribute to sleeping problems. Predisposing factors relate to issues that commonly increase an individual's risk of developing sleep problems—such as old age, having an anxious-prone personality, and a family history of insomnia—and often have no connection to patients' current illnesses. Precipitating factors relate to sleep problem triggers that may be more specific to patients' illnesses—such as hospitalization, medication (e.g., opioids, corticosteroids), cancer treatments that affect sleep, and cancer-related symptoms (e.g., pain, dyspnoea). Perpetuating factors maintain or worsen patients' sleep problems over time and include unhelpful behaviours, such as excessive daytime napping and maladaptive cognitions related to sleep (Jakobsen et al., 2022).

The sleep problems of patients in palliative care may be treated with medication and nonpharmaceutical methods. Despite the efficacy of evidence-based medications in the general population, it remains uncertain whether these medications are equally effective and safe for patients with cancer. A study by Howell et al. (2014) illustrates that when prescribing sleep medication for patients in palliative care, the patient's preference, possible side effects (e.g., nausea, dependence), comorbidities, concurrent drug reactions, and contraindications need to be considered. In terms of the nonpharmaceutical approach, patients in palliative care may benefit from non-medication methods, such as cognitive behavioural interventions (Bernatchez et al., 2019; Kwekkeboom et al., 2018). Exercise and mindfulness-based stress reduction therapy are also potentially helpful in addressing cancer-related sleep issues (Matthews & Wang, 2022). However, a certain portion of patients under palliative care may not be able to actively engage in these nonpharmacological approaches (Hajjar, 2008), thereby reducing the positive impact of the treatment above other approaches for sleep problems.

In addition, barriers exist that limit the effectiveness of treatment for sleep problems among patients in palliative care. A study by Khater et al. (2019) finds that although the majority (70%) of patients with cancer report having poor sleep quality problems, these are often not assessed during hospitalization. Only 8% of cancer patients who report sleep problems to a nurse have received interventions aimed at promoting better sleep. Patients may be reluctant to disclose their sleep problems or seek solutions because they believe the medical team is too busy to handle such issues or that their sleep issues are normal or are temporary reactions to their illness and/or treatments received. Sleep problems often appear to be overlooked and inadequately managed, and they remain an unmet need among this vulnerable population.

Negative Impact of Unmet Physical Needs

Unmet physical needs, including pain, fatigue, and sleep problems, appear to be highly prevalent. Despite evidence-based practice, practical barriers (limited treatment options) and patient-related barriers (e.g., under-reporting of needs, misconceptions) may limit the effectiveness of pharmaceutical and nonpharmaceutical interventions. Without effective management, unmet physical needs would negatively impact the quality of end-of-life. Physically, these unmet needs may exacerbate the symptoms of illness, such as pain, nausea, and vomiting, or increase their frequency (Mercadante et al., 2015). Socially, unmet physical needs may result in reduced social interactions and decreased participation in social activities (Scott et al., 2011). Cognitively, patients may encounter difficulties with concentration and thinking (Bennett et al., 2007). Psychologically, patients may often experience more negative emotions (e.g., frustration, irritability) and a higher risk of anxiety and depression (Delgado-Guay et al., 2011; Scott et al., 2011). Hence, innovative and alternative approaches are needed to address the physical needs that have been unaddressed by traditional interventions.

Unmet Psychological Needs

"I cannot do what I used to do now."

Reduced Autonomy

Houska and Loučka (2019) define autonomy in patients under palliative care as actively living a normal life while facing death. These authors identify two core domains of autonomy at the end-of-life stage: being normal and taking charge. *Being normal* involves perceiving the body as being normal despite experiencing physical changes due to illness symptoms (e.g., pain, dyspnoea, weight loss) and disease progression. What activity matters depends on the patient's understanding of autonomy, which can include continuing daily activities, living in the present, and making meaningful plans. *Taking charge* involves perceiving the self as a whole individual, being treated with respect and trust, and not burdening the family. It also involves patients being able to manage their end-of-life process in terms of issues such as making decisions and meeting their own needs. However, the significance of autonomy for patients in palliative care is often overlooked or misunderstood for two reasons (Houska & Loučka, 2019). First, there is a widespread belief that autonomy is limited to a person's rational and independent decision-making. Second, patients in palliative care are often perceived as being passive recipients of care; and the possible contribution of the patient themself is overlooked. Consequently, patients in palliative care continue to experience unfulfilled autonomy needs.

Depression

Depression is characterized by persistent feelings of sadness or loss of interest accompanied by various symptoms, such as changes in appetite, sleep disturbances, fatigue, feelings of worthlessness, and difficulty concentrating, which significantly impair daily functioning (American Psychiatric Association, 2013). Depression is not uncommon in palliative care. A meta-analysis by Mitchell et al. (2011) reports that approximately one in four patients in palliative care experience depression. Similarly, a literature review by Miovic and Block (2007) reveals that 5% to 26% of patients with advanced cancer meet the criteria for major depression. Depression is found to be associated with a higher likelihood of hastening death wishes and suicidal risk among patients in palliative care (Noorani & Montagnini, 2007).

Depression or low mood is a psychological problem that necessitates immediate attention in palliative care. However, medical professionals often overlook such issues among palliative care patients, which often results in untreated mood problems. There are several reasons why depression or low mood might not be identified. First, palliative care patients may perceive depression as a sign of weakness and be reluctant to talk to others about their symptoms. Second, medical professionals may find it challenging to differentiate between clinical depression and normal adjustment reactions to approaching death, such as sadness or anticipatory grief. They may also encounter difficulties in conducting thorough assessments of patients' psychological experiences due to time constraints or concerns about evoking negative emotions in patients. Lastly, there is a lack of consensus among existing studies on the most effective treatment approaches in this vulnerable population, while non-medication approaches are not well supported by empirical studies (Noorani & Montagnini, 2007; Perusinghe et al., 2021). Depression therefore appears to be an unmet need that warrants immediate attention.

Anxiety

Patients with terminal illnesses may experience anxiety or fear related to cancer and its physical symptoms (Penman & Ellis, 2015). This includes worrying about the spread or recurrence of cancer, physical suffering, deterioration of one's abilities, lack of control over one's physical condition, and poor disease progression. Furthermore, anxiety or fear can be associated with one's relationship with the self and others, such as anxiety about dying alone, feelings of emptiness, and the impact of their illness on loved ones (Penman & Ellis, 2015). Hence, anxiety appears to be another prevalent psychological need observed in patients under palliative care. According to a systematic review by Wang et al. (2018), 15% to 42% of advanced cancer patients consider anxiety to be an unmet care need. A longitudinal observation of anxiety among palliative care cancer patients (Sewtz et al., 2021) summarizes that the prevalence of anxiety ranges from 11% to 63%. The findings of these studies underscore the significant need to address anxiety among patients with terminal illnesses.

Although anxiety can have a significant impact on patients' well-being, anxiety management is challenging in palliative care settings. The results of a cross-sectional survey (Atkin et al., 2017) reveal a lack of robust evidence regarding the assessment and management of anxiety in palliative care, particularly for pharmaceutical approaches. It is also difficult to access nonpharmaceutical interventions in a timely fashion. Atkin et al. (2017) also find that the majority of doctors encounter difficulties in distinguishing pathological anxiety from reasonable worries towards end-of-life. As such, anxiety continues to be an unaddressed need for patients under palliative care.

Negative Impact of Unmet Psychological Needs

Unmet psychological needs such as reduced autonomy, depression, and anxiety can negatively impact well-being. Studies have shown that depression is associated with poor adherence to cancer treatment, lower cancer survival, and an increased risk of suicide (Pitman et al., 2018). Patients with depression or anxiety exhibit reduced social functioning, more disability, and greater overall functional impairment than patients without depression or anxiety (Katon, 2003). In patients with advanced cancer, depression and anxiety have been associated with decreased cognitive functioning (Mystakidou et al., 2005; Smith et al., 2003), poor adherence to prescribed treatment regimens (DiMatteo et al., 2000), and limited personal self-efficacy (Institute of Medicine, 2008). Anxiety is also related to a greater frequency of nausea, pain, and dyspnoea (Delgado-Guay et al., 2009). In short, unmet psychological needs significantly reduce the quality of life of patients, and innovative interventions are required to address these unmet needs.

Unmet Social Needs

"I don't have someone to talk to now."

Social Isolation

Social isolation refers to the lack of social connections with family, friends, or the community (Ritchie & Kotwal, 2023). The results of a cross-sectional study (Kotwal et al., 2021) show that over one-fourth of individuals in their last three months of life experience social isolation. Two factors lead to social isolation in palliative care settings (Ritchie & Kotwal, 2023). First, structural and community-level factors, such as transportation barriers and technological constraints, restrict the access of patients to social opportunities. Second, patient-related factors, such as poor physical health, reduced independence, limited mobility, and embarrassment due to a lack of control over one's symptoms (Fitzsimons et al., 2007). Socioemotional selectivity theory (Carstensen, 1992) proposes that at the end-of-life stage, patients tend to limit their social circle to a few significant others, such as immediate family members or confidants, as they are more conscious of the limited time they have left. This narrowing of the social circle implies fewer opportunities for social interaction and fewer sources of social support. Thus, structural and community-level factors, as well as patient-related factors, appear to bar patients from social interaction, which leaves social isolation as an unmet social need.

Inadequate Emotional Support

Wenrich et al. (2003) identify three levels of emotional support in the context of terminal illness. The first level is to provide emotional support through compassion, warmth, and care. The second level involves being responsive to patients' emotional needs, fostering hope, and maintaining a positive attitude. The third level involves taking an active role in the patient's life and offering comfort. Understanding and love are considered to be foundational elements in emotional support for patients who are faced with existential challenges.

Similar to emotional and psychological needs, some relational and communicative barriers may hinder patients' access to emotional needs (Nagelschmidt et al., 2021). For example, patients with traditional hierarchical roles or values within the family or society may be reluctant to share their existential distress or concerns. Patients' families and friends may also feel uncertain about what to say or how to offer adequate and appropriate emotional support to patients (LeSeure & Chongkham-Ang, 2015; Salander & Spetz, 2002). Furthermore, healthcare professionals who provide emotional support may experience compassion fatigue and burnout (Lin & Fan, 2020). These factors contribute to the unmet need for emotional support among patients in palliative care settings.

Negative Impact of Unmet Social Needs

Unmet social needs, such as social isolation and lack of emotional support, can significantly compromise the well-being of patients under palliative care. Without sufficient social support, patients may experience worsening physical symptoms (e.g., pain and fatigue), cognitive and physical decline, and increased mortality rates (Ritchie & Kotwal, 2023). In addition, a lack of social connection and emotional support may hinder the patient's ability to fulfil their end-of-life goals (Kotwal et al., 2021). Emotionally, inadequate social support may leave patients feeling isolated, misunderstood, and disconnected from others, which may lead to a sense of hopelessness and a higher risk of developing depression (Somasundaram & Devamani, 2016). These negative impacts are consistent with the findings of Azevedo et al. (2017), who highlight a significant association between inadequate social support and lower overall quality of life in patients. This emphasizes the urgency and importance of addressing unmet social needs with an innovative approach.

Unmet Spiritual Needs

"I can't see the meaning of living now."

Meaning in Life

Spirituality is an aspect of human life that touches on the way a person experiences, expresses, and/or seeks meaning, purpose, and transcendence, and the way they connect to the moment, to self, and/or to others (Nolan et al., 2011). Specifically, meaning in life refers to a person's subjective understanding of his/her purpose in life and the importance of that purpose to him/her. It comprises both cognitive and emotional components (Fegg et al., 2016). The cognitive component consists of elements such as values, beliefs, and goals that serve as a framework for one's existence. The emotional component brings a sense of fulfilment and the motivation to actively participate in life experiences. The phenomenon of meaning in life can be explained by the terror management theory (Carreno & Eisenbeck, 2022; Greenberg & Arndt, 2012). The theory states that fear and anxiety triggered by reminders of mortality may elicit adaptive responses (such as acceptance and searching for meaning) and maladaptive responses (such as denial and avoidance). The importance of considering perceived meaning in life among patients in palliative care is reflected in Bernard et al.'s (2017) study, which explores the relationships among spiritual, existential, and psychological needs in patients. The study finds that patients with lower levels of meaning in life tend to experience more psychological distress; this indicates the impact of this need.

Pearce et al.'s (2012) study on unmet spiritual care needs in advanced cancer patients indicates that 28% of patients do not receive the level of spiritual care they desire despite healthcare professionals having already been involved to lessen the negative impact of mortality reminders. A common barrier to meeting patients' spiritual needs is their uncontrolled physical symptoms, which often overshadow the need for meaning in life (Laranjeira et al., 2023).

Negative Impact of Meaninglessness in Life

Research has shown that meaninglessness in life may impede the overall well-being of patients in palliative care. Patients without meaning in life may be unable to manage illnesses effectively, are less tolerant of physical symptoms, and encounter more sleep and interpersonal problems (Guerrero-Torrelles et al., 2017; Kleftaras & Psarra, 2012). A cross-sectional study on cancer patients (Testoni et al., 2018) reports that a lower level of meaning in life is associated with higher levels of psychological distress, anxiety, and depression. Patients with lower-level meaning in life are more likely to report higher levels of demoralization, disengagement, and hastening death wishes (Guerrero-Torrelles et al., 2017). A possible explanation for this is that when a patient's life lacks meaning for them, they may be more dissatisfied with their life overall and encounter more difficulties accomplishing their life objectives. This can result in emptiness, stagnation, and an overall dissatisfaction with life (Kleftaras & Psarra, 2012). Unmet spiritual needs may undermine the quality of patients' end-of-life, and alternate approaches are needed in offering meaningful spiritual support that is otherwise unaddressed by traditional interventions.

Other Needs

Inadequate Advance Care Planning

Advance care planning (ACP) is indispensable in palliative care. ACP refers to a proactive communication process that involves the patient and their healthcare providers, family members, and caregivers to determine the appropriate care for the patient in advance (Hospital Authority, 2019). Facilitating open discussions about ACP promotes greater alignment in care preferences, reduces aggressive medical interventions at end-of-life, and enhances the patient's quality of life. In contrast, the inability to openly discuss end-of-life issues may result in psychological challenges, such as negative feelings, a sense of uncertainty, and diminished control among patients in palliative care (Nagelschmidt et al., 2021). Therefore, ACP is considered to be essential in patient-centred care.

Despite the benefits of ACP, emotional and cognitive barriers may hinder the ACP process. Emotionally, patients and their families/caregivers may feel overwhelmed by disease symptoms and progression and, thus, be too emotionally stressed for discussions about ACP. The desire to protect loved ones from difficult emotions, and concerns about evoking psychological distress, may also discourage patients and family members from participating in ACP. In addition, cognitively, some patients in palliative care may have limited awareness and knowledge of ACP, while others may find the concept of ACP too abstract and difficult to comprehend (Kim & Flieger, 2023; Nagelschmidt et al., 2021). These factors may prevent proactive engagement in ACP, leaving ACP as an unmet need in palliative care.

Inadequate Support for Palliative Care Providers

Palliative care providers are healthcare workers who work in palliative care settings; these providers include but are not limited to doctors, nurses, and allied health professionals. However, there appears to be little psychological or emotional support available for these healthcare professionals. According to a meta-analysis by Gómez-Urquiza et al. (2020), 24% of palliative care nurses report high levels of emotional exhaustion, while a systematic review by Parola et al. (2017) finds that 17% of health professionals in palliative care experience burnout. These findings highlight the urgency and importance of considering the psychological well-being of palliative care providers.

If palliative care providers receive insufficient emotional support, the quality of patient care may be compromised. Palliative care providers are no different than medical professionals in other settings, who face everyday workplace stressors such as heavy workloads and long working hours. In addition, palliative care providers may face unique challenges, such as frequently encountering death, witnessing patients' suffering, and having to break bad news to patients and their families. All these factors may contribute to suboptimal psychological well-being among palliative care providers, leading to higher rates of staff sickness and absence, potentially compromised patient safety due to more medical errors and poorer patient care (Papworth et al., 2023; Hall et al., 2016).

Conclusions

This chapter has shed light on the significant unmet needs of patients in palliative care, emphasizing the profound impact these deficiencies can have on their physical, psychological, social, and spiritual well-being. Despite advancements in evidence-based practices, a portion of patients still struggle with unrelieved pain, emotional distress, social isolation, and a sense of spiritual emptiness, all of which can diminish their quality of life. Fortunately, alternative interventions supported by advanced technology, such as VR, bring new hope. The following chapters explore the use of VR, looking into its theoretical foundation and possible clinical applications in palliative care, which showcase its immense potential to fulfil the unmet needs identified in this chapter.

References

American Psychiatric Association. (2013). *Diagnostic and statistical manual of mental disorders* (5th ed.). https://doi.org/10.1176/appi.books.9780890425596

Anekar, A. A., Hendrix, J. M., & Cascella, M. (2023). WHO analgesic ladder. In *StatPearls [Internet]*. StatPearls Publishing. https://www.ncbi.nlm.nih.gov/books/NBK554435/

Atkin, N., Vickerstaff, V., & Candy, B. (2017). "Worried to death": The assessment and management of anxiety in patients with advanced life-limiting disease, a national survey of palliative medicine physicians. *BMC Palliative Care, 16*(1), 69. https://doi.org/10.1186/s12904-017-0245-5

Azevedo, C., Pessalacia, J. D. R., Mata, L. R. F. D, Zoboli, E. L. C. P., & Pereira, M. D G. (2017). Interface between social support, quality of life and depression in users eligible for palliative care. *Revista Da Escola de Enfermagem Da U S P, 51*, e03245. https://doi.org/10.1590/S1980-220X2016038003245

Azevedo São Leão Ferreira, K., Kimura, M., & Jacobsen Teixeira, M. (2006). The WHO analgesic ladder for cancer pain control, twenty years of use. How much pain relief does one get from using it? *Supportive Care in Cancer, 14*(11), 1086–1093. https://doi.org/10.1007/s00520-006-0086-x

Bennett, B., Goldstein, D., Friedlander, M., Hickie, I., & Lloyd, A. (2007). The experience of cancer-related fatigue and chronic fatigue syndrome: A qualitative and comparative study. *Journal of Pain and Symptom Management, 34*(2), 126–135. https://doi.org/10.1016/j.jpainsymman.2006.10.014

Bennett, S., Pigott, A., Beller, E. M., Haines, T., Meredith, P., & Delaney, C. (2016). Educational interventions for the management of cancer-related fatigue in adults. *Cochrane Database of Systematic Reviews, 11*(11), CD008144. https://doi.org/10.1002/14651858.CD008144.pub2

Berger, A. M., Mooney, K., Alvarez-Perez, A., Breitbart, W. S., Carpenter, K. M., Cella, D., Cleeland, C., Dotan, E., Eisenberger, M. A., Escalante, C. P., Jacobsen, P. B., Jankowski, C., LeBlanc, T., Ligibel, J. A., Loggers, E. T., Mandrell, B., Murphy, B. A., Palesh, O., Pirl, W. F., . . . National Comprehensive Cancer Network. (2015). Cancer-related fatigue, version 2.2015. *Journal of the National Comprehensive Cancer Network, 13*(8), 1012–1039.

Bernard, M., Strasser, F., Gamondi, C., Braunschweig, G., Forster, M., Kaspers-Elekes, K., Walther Veri, S., Borasio, G. D., Pralong, G., Pralong, J., Marthy, S., Soloni, C., Bisi, C., & Magaya, N. K. (2017). Relationship between spirituality, meaning in life, psychological distress, wish for hastened death, and their influence on quality of life in palliative care patients. *Journal of Pain and Symptom Management, 54*(4), 514–522. https://doi.org/10.1016/j.jpainsymman.2017.07.019

Bernatchez, M. S., Savard, J., Savard, M.-H., & Aubin, M. (2019). Feasibility of a cognitive-behavioral and environmental intervention for sleep-wake difficulties in community-dwelling cancer patients receiving palliative care. *Cancer Nursing, 42*(5), 396–409. https://doi.org/10.1097/NCC.0000000000000603

Borneman, T. (2013). Assessment and management of cancer-related fatigue. *Journal of Hospice and Palliative Nursing, 15*(2), 77–86. https://doi.org/10.1097/NJH.0b013e318286dc19

Carreno, D. F., & Eisenbeck, N. (2022). Existential insights in cancer: Meaning in life adaptability. *Medicina, 58*(4), 461.

Carstensen, L. L. (1992, September). Social and emotional patterns in adulthood: Support for socioemotional selectivity theory. *Psychology and Aging, 7*(3), 331–338. https://doi.org/10.1037/0882-7974.7.3.331

Corbett, T. K., Groarke, A., Devane, D., Carr, J., Walsh, J. C., & McGuire, B. E. (2019). The effectiveness of psychological interventions for fatigue in cancer survivors: Systematic review of randomised controlled trials. *Systematic Reviews, 8*(1), 324. https://doi.org/10.1186/s13643-019-1230-2

Dean, A. (2019). The holistic management of fatigue within palliative care. *International Journal of Palliative Nursing, 25*(8), 368–376. https://doi.org/10.12968/ijpn.2019.25.8.368

Delgado-Guay, M., Parsons, H. A., Li, Z., Palmer, J. L., & Bruera, E. (2009). Symptom distress in advanced cancer patients with anxiety and depression in the palliative care setting. *Supportive Care in Cancer: Official Journal of the Multinational Association of Supportive Care in Cancer, 17*(5), 573–579. https://doi.org/10.1007/s00520-008-0529-7

Delgado-Guay, M., Yennurajalingam, S., Parsons, H., Palmer, J. L., & Bruera, E. (2011). Association between self-reported sleep disturbance and other symptoms in patients with advanced cancer. *Journal of Pain and Symptom Management, 41*(5), 819–827. https://doi.org/10.1016/j.jpainsymman.2010.07.015

DiMatteo, M. R., Lepper, H. S., & Croghan, T. W. (2000). Depression is a risk factor for noncompliance with medical treatment: Meta-analysis of the effects of anxiety and depression on patient adherence. *Archives of Internal Medicine (1960), 160*(14), 2101–2107. https://doi.org/10.1001/archinte.160.14.2101

Dobratz, M. C. (2009). Word choices of advanced cancer patients: Frequency of nociceptive and neuropathic pain. *American Journal of Hospice & Palliative Medicine, 25*(6), 469–475. https://doi.org/10.1177/1049909108322293

Fegg, M., Kudla, D., Brandstätter, M., Deffner, V., & Küchenhoff, H. (2016). Individual meaning in life assessed with the schedule for meaning in life evaluation: Toward a circumplex meaning model. *Palliative & Supportive Care, 14*(2), 91–98. https://doi.org/10.1017/S1478951515000656

Fitzsimons, D., Mullan, D., Wilson, J. S., Conway, B., Corcoran, B., Dempster, M., Gamble, J., Stewart, C., Rafferty, S., McMahon, M., MacMahon, J., Mulholland, P., Stockdale, P., Chew, E., Hanna, L., Brown, J., Ferguson, G., & Fogarty, D. (2007). The challenge of patients' unmet palliative care needs in the final stages of chronic illness. *Palliative Medicine, 21*(4), 313–322. https://doi.org/10.1177/0269216307077711

Fuller, J. T., Hartland, M. C., Maloney, L. T., & Davison, K. (2018). Therapeutic effects of aerobic and resistance exercises for cancer survivors: A systematic review of meta-analyses of clinical trials. *British Journal of Sports Medicine, 52*(20), 1311. https://doi.org/10.1136/bjsports-2017-098285

Gómez-Urquiza, J. L., Albendín-García, L., Velando-Soriano, A., Ortega-Campos, E., Ramírez-Baena, L., Membrive-Jiménez, M. J., & Suleiman-Martos, N. (2020). Burnout in palliative care nurses, prevalence and risk factors: A systematic review with meta-analysis. *International Journal of Environmental Research and Public Health, 17*(20), 7672. https://doi.org/10.3390/ijerph17207672

Greenberg, J., & Arndt, J. (2012). Terror management theory. In P. A. M. van Lange, A. W. Kruglanski, & E. T. Higgins (Eds.), *Handbook of theories of social psychology* (Vol. 1, pp. 398–415). SAGE Publications Ltd.

Guerrero-Torrelles, M., Monforte-Royo, C., Tomás-Sábado, J., Marimon, F., Porta-Sales, J., & Balaguer, A. (2017). Meaning in life as a mediator between physical impairment and the wish to hasten death in patients with advanced cancer. *Journal of Pain and Symptom Management*, *54*(6), 826–834. https://doi.org/10.1016/j.jpainsymman.2017.04.018

Hajjar, R. R. (2008). Sleep disturbance in palliative care. *Clinics in Geriatric Medicine*, *24*(1), 83–91. https://doi.org/10.1016/j.cger.2007.08.003

Hall, L. H., Johnson, J., Watt, I., Tsipa, A., & O'Connor, D. B. (2016). Healthcare staff wellbeing, burnout, and patient safety: A systematic review. *PloS One*, *11*(7), e0159015. https://doi.org/10.1371/journal.pone.0159015

Hospital Authority. (2019). *HA guidelines on advance care planning*. Patient Safety & Risk Management Department/Quality & Safety Division. https://www.ha.org.hk/haho/ho/psrm/EACPGuidelines.pdf

Houska, A., & Loučka, M. (2019). Patients' autonomy at the end of life: A critical review. *Journal of Pain and Symptom Management*, *57*(4), 835–845. https://doi.org/10.1016/j.jpainsymman.2018.12.339

Howell, D., Oliver, T. K., Keller-Olaman, S., Davidson, J. R., Garland, S., Samuels, C., Savard, J., Harris, C., Aubin, M., Olson, K., Sussman, J., MacFarlane, J., & Taylor, C. (2014). Sleep disturbance in adults with cancer: A systematic review of evidence for best practices in assessment and management for clinical practice. *Annals of Oncology*, *25*(4), 791–800. https://doi.org/10.1093/annonc/mdt506

Institute of Medicine. (2008). *Cancer care for the whole patient: Meeting psychosocial concerns*. The National Academic Press.

Jacobsen, R., Møldrup, C., Christrup, L., & Sjøgren, P. (2009). Patient-related barriers to cancer pain management: A systematic exploratory review. *Scandinavian Journal of Caring Sciences*, *23*(1), 190–208. https://doi.org/10.1111/j.1471-6712.2008.00601.x

Jakobsen, G., Gjeilo, K. H., Hjermstad, M. J., & Klepstad, P. (2022). An update on prevalence, assessment, and risk factors for sleep disturbances in patients with advanced cancer—implications for health care providers and clinical research. *Cancers*, *14*(16), 3933. https://doi.org/10.3390/cancers14163933

Katon, W. J. (2003). Clinical and health services relationships between major depression, depressive symptoms, and general medical illness. *Biological Psychiatry (1969)*, *54*(3), 216–226. https://doi.org/10.1016/S0006-3223(03)00273-7

Khater, W., Masha'al, D., & al-Sayaheen, A. (2019). Sleep assessment and interventions for patients living with cancer from the patients' and nurses' perspective. *International Journal of Palliative Nursing*, *25*(7), 316–324. https://doi.org/10.12968/ijpn.2019.25.7.316

Kim, H., & Flieger, S. P. (2023). Barriers to effective communication about advance care planning and palliative care: A qualitative study. *Journal of Hospice and Palliative Care*, *26*(2), 42–50. https://doi.org/10.14475/jhpc.2023.26.2.42

Kleftaras, G., & Psarra, E. (2012). Meaning in life, psychological well-being and depressive symptomatology: A comparative study. *Psychology*, *3*, 337–345.

Kotwal, A. A., Cenzer, I. S., Waite, L. J., Covinsky, K. E., Perissinotto, C. M., Boscardin, W. J., Hawkley, L. C., Dale, W., & Smith, A. K. (2021). The epidemiology of social isolation and loneliness among older adults during the last years of life. *Journal of the American Geriatrics Society (JAGS)*, *69*(11), 3081–3091. https://doi.org/10.1111/jgs.17366

Kwekkeboom, K., Zhang, Y., Campbell, T., Coe, C. L., Costanzo, E., Serlin, R. C., & Ward, S. (2018). Randomized controlled trial of a brief cognitive-behavioral strategies intervention for the pain, fatigue, and sleep disturbance symptom cluster in advanced cancer. *Psycho-Oncology (Chichester, England)*, 27(12), 2761–2769. https://doi.org/10.1002/pon.4883

Laranjeira, C., Dixe, M. A., & Querido, A. (2023). Perceived barriers to providing spiritual care in palliative care among professionals: A portuguese cross-sectional study. *International Journal of Environmental Research and Public Health*, 20(12), 6121. https://doi.org/10.3390/ijerph20126121

Leppert, W., Zajaczkowska, R., Wordliczek, J., Dobrogowski, J., Woron, J., & Krzakowski, M. (2016). Pathophysiology and clinical characteristics of pain in most common locations in cancer patients. *J Physiol Pharmacol*, 67(6), 787–799.

LeSeure, P., & Chongkham-Ang, S. (2015). The experience of caregivers living with cancer patients: A systematic review and meta-synthesis. *Journal of Personalized Medicine*, 5(4), 406–439. https://doi.org/10.3390/jpm5040406

Lin, W. C., & Fan, S. Y. (2020). Emotional and cognitive barriers of bereavement care among clinical staff in hospice palliative care. *Palliative & Supportive Care*, 18(6), 676–682. https://doi.org/10.1017/S147895152000022X

Matthews, E. E., & Wang, S. Y. (2022, February). Cancer-related sleep wake disturbances. In *Seminars in oncology nursing* (Vol. 38, No. 1, p. 151253). WB Saunders.

Mercadante, S., Aielli, F., Adile, C., Ferrera, P., Valle, A., Cartoni, C., Pizzuto, M., Caruselli, A., Parsi, R., Cortegiani, A., Masedu, F., Valenti, M., Ficorella, C., & Porzio, G. (2015). Sleep disturbances in patients with advanced cancer in different palliative care settings. *Journal of Pain and Symptom Management*, 50(6), 786–792. https://doi.org/10.1016/j.jpainsymman.2015.06.018

Miovic, M., & Block, S. (2007). Psychiatric disorders in advanced cancer. *Cancer*, 110(8), 1665–1676. https://doi.org/10.1002/cncr.22980

Mitchell, A. J., Chan, M., Bhatti, H., Halton, M., Grassi, L., Johansen, C., & Meader, N. (2011). Prevalence of depression, anxiety, and adjustment disorder in oncological, haematological, and palliative-care settings: A meta-analysis of 94 interview-based studies. *The Lancet Oncology*, 12(2), 160–174. https://doi.org/10.1016/S1470-2045(11)70002-X

Mystakidou, K., Tsilika, E., Parpa, E., Katsouda, E., Galanos, A., & Vlahos, L. (2005). Assessment of anxiety and depression in advanced cancer patients and their relationship with quality of life. *Quality of Life Research*, 14(8), 1825–1833. https://doi.org/10.1007/s11136-005-4324-3

Nagelschmidt, K., Leppin, N., Seifart, C., Rief, W., & von Blanckenburg, P. (2021). Systematic mixed-method review of barriers to end-of-life communication in the family context. *BMJ Supportive & Palliative Care*, 11(3), 253–263. https://doi.org/10.1136/bmjspcare-2020-002219

Nolan, S., Saltmarsh, P., & Leget, C. J. W. (2011). Spiritual care in palliative care: Working towards an EAPC task force. *European Journal of Palliative Care*, 86–89.

Noorani, N. H., & Montagnini, M. (2007). Recognizing depression in palliative care patients. *Journal of Palliative Medicine*, 10(2), 458–464. https://doi.org/10.1089/jpm.2006.0099

Nzwalo, I., Aboim, M. A., Joaquim, N., Marreiros, A., & Nzwalo, H. (2020). Systematic review of the prevalence, predictors, and treatment of insomnia in palliative care. *American Journal of Hospice and Palliative Medicine*, 37(11), 957–969. https://doi.org/10.1177/1049909120907021

Papworth, A., Ziegler, L., Beresford, B., Mukherjee, S., Fraser, L., Fisher, V., O'Neill, M., Golder, S., Bedendo, A., & Taylor, J. (2023). Psychological well-being of hospice staff: Systematic review. *BMJ Supportive & Palliative Care*, 13(e3), e597–e611. https://doi.org/10.1136/spcare-2022-004012

Parola, V., Coelho, A., Cardoso, D., Sandgren, A., & Apóstolo, J. (2017). Prevalence of burnout in health professionals working in palliative care: A systematic review. *JBI Database of Systematic Reviews and Implementation Reports*, *15*(7), 1905–1933. https://doi.org/10.11124/jbisrir-2016-003309

Pearce, M. J., Coan, A. D., Herndon, J. E., Koenig, H. G., & Abernethy, A. P. (2012). Unmet spiritual care needs impact emotional and spiritual well-being in advanced cancer patients. *Supportive Care in Cancer*, *20*(10), 2269–2276. https://doi.org/10.1007/s00520-011-1335-1

Penman, J., & Ellis, B. (2015). Palliative care clients' and caregivers' notion of fear and their strategies for overcoming it. *Palliative & Supportive Care*, *13*(3), 777–785. https://doi.org/10.1017/S1478951514000571

Perusinghe, M., Chen, K. Y., & McDermott, B. (2021). Evidence-based management of depression in palliative care: A systematic review. *Journal of Palliative Medicine*, *24*(5), 767–781. https://doi.org/10.1089/jpm.2020.0659

Pitman, A., Suleman, S., Hyde, N., & Hodgkiss, A. (2018). Depression and anxiety in patients with cancer. *BMJ (Online)*, *361*, k1415. https://doi.org/10.1136/bmj.k1415

Radbruch, L., Strasser, F., Elsner, F., Gonçalves, J. F., Løge, J., Kaasa, S., Nauck, F., & Stone, P. (2008). Fatigue in palliative care patients—an EAPC approach. *Palliative Medicine*, *22*(1), 13–32. https://doi.org/10.1177/0269216307085183

Ritchie, C. S., & Kotwal, A. A. (2023). Loneliness and social isolation in palliative care: A call to action. *Journal of Palliative Medicine*, *26*(8), 1032–1034. https://doi.org/10.1089/jpm.2023.0425

Salander, P., & Spetz, A. (2002). How do patients and spouses deal with the serious facts of malignant glioma? *Palliative Medicine*, *16*(4), 305–313. https://doi.org/10.1191/0269216302pm569oa

Savard, J., & Morin, C. M. (2001). Insomnia in the context of cancer: A review of a neglected problem. *Journal of Clinical Oncology: Official Journal of the American Society of Clinical Oncology*, *19*(3), 895–908. https://doi.org/10.1200/JCO.2001.19.3.895

Scott, J. A., Lasch, K. E., Barsevick, A. M., & Piault-Louis, E. (2011). Patients' experiences with cancer-related fatigue: A review and synthesis of qualitative research. *Oncology Nursing Forum*, *38*(3), E191–E203. https://doi.org/10.1188/11.ONF.E191-E203

Sewtz, C., Muscheites, W., Grosse-Thie, C., Kriesen, U., Leithaeuser, M., Glaeser, D., Hansen, P., Kundt, G., Fuellen, G., & Junghanss, C. (2021). Longitudinal observation of anxiety and depression among palliative care cancer patients. *Annals of Palliative Medicine*, *10*(4), 3836–3846. https://doi.org/10.21037/apm-20-1346

Shun, S.-C., Hsiao, F.-H., & Lai, Y.-H. (2011). Relationship between hope and fatigue characteristics in newly diagnosed outpatients with cancer. *Oncology Nursing Forum*, *38*(2), E81–E86. https://doi.org/10.1188/11.ONF.E81-E86

Shun, S.-C., Lai, Y., & Hsiao, F. (2009). Patient-related barriers to fatigue communication in cancer patients receiving active treatment. *The Oncologist (Dayton, Ohio)*, *14*(9), 936–943. https://doi.org/10.1634/theoncologist.2009-0048

Smith, E., Gomm, S., & Dickens, C. (2003). Assessing the independent contribution to quality of life from anxiety and depression in patients with advanced cancer. *Palliative Medicine*, *17*(6), 509–513. https://doi.org/10.1191/0269216303pm781oa

Somasundaram, R. O., & Devamani, K. A. (2016). A comparative study on resilience, perceived social support and hopelessness among cancer patients treated with curative and palliative care. *Indian Journal of Palliative Care*, 22(2), 135–140. https://doi.org/10.4103/0973-1075.179606

Spielman, A. J., Caruso, L. S., & Glovinsky, P. B. (1987). A behavioral perspective on insomnia treatment. *The Psychiatric clinics of North America*, 10(4), 541–553.

Stone, P., Richardson, A., Ream, E., Smith, A. G., Kerr, D. J., & Kearney, N. (2000). Cancer-related fatigue: Inevitable, unimportant and untreatable? Results of a multi-centre patient survey. *Annals of Oncology*, 11(8), 971–975. https://doi. org/10.1023/A:1008318932641

Testoni, I., Sansonetto, G., Ronconi, L., Rodelli, M., Baracco, G., & Grassi, L. (2018). Meaning of life, representation of death, and their association with psychological distress. *Palliative & Supportive Care*, 16(5), 511–519. https://doi. org/10.1017/S1478951517000669

van den Beuken-van Everdingen, M. H. J., Hochstenbach, L. M. J., Joosten, E. A. J., Tjan-Heijnen, V. C. G., & Janssen, D. J. A. (2016). Update on prevalence of pain in patients with cancer: Systematic review and meta-analysis. *Journal of Pain and Symptom Management*, 51(6), 1070–1090.e9. https://doi.org/10.1016/j. jpainsymman.2015.12.340

Wang, T., Molassiotis, A., Chung, B. P. M., & Tan, J.-Y. (2018). Unmet care needs of advanced cancer patients and their informal caregivers: A systematic review. *BMC Palliative Care*, 17(1), 96. https://doi.org/10.1186/s12904-018-0346-9

Wang, T., Molassiotis, A., Tan, J.-Y., Chung, B. P. M., & Huang, H.-Q. (2021). Prevalence and correlates of unmet palliative care needs in dyads of Chinese patients with advanced cancer and their informal caregivers: A cross-sectional survey. *Supportive Care in Cancer*, 29(3), 1683–1698. https://doi.org/10.1007/s00520-020-05657-w

Wenrich, M. D., Curtis, J. R., Ambrozy, D. A., Carline, J. D., Shannon, S. E., & Ramsey, P. G. (2003). Dying patients' need for emotional support and personalized care from physicians: Perspectives of patients with terminal illness, families, and health care providers. *Journal of Pain and Symptom Management*, 25(3), 236–246. https://doi.org/10.1016/S0885-3924(02)00694-2

Wilkie, D. J., & Ezenwa, M. O. (2012). Pain and symptom management in palliative care and at end of life. *Nursing Outlook*, 60(6), 357–364. https://doi. org/10.1016/j.outlook.2012.08.002

Yavuzsen, T., Davis, M. P., Ranganathan, V. K., Walsh, D., Siemionow, V., Kirkova, J., Khoshknabi, D., Lagman, R., LeGrand, S., & Yue, G. H. (2009). Cancer-related fatigue: Central or peripheral? *Journal of Pain and Symptom Management*, 38(4), 587–596. https://doi.org/10.1016/j.jpainsymman.2008.12.003

Section II

Theoretical Foundation for the Use of Virtual Reality

This section provides a comprehensive overview of VR, its therapeutic potential in palliative care, and the possible theoretical basis that informs its use. Chapter 4 introduces VR technology, discussing its development, important concepts such as presence and immersion, and application in healthcare. Chapter 5 examines the specific application of VR in palliative care, showcasing its emerging evidence supporting its efficacy in addressing patients' biopsychosocial–spiritual needs and other relevant needs. Chapter 6 explores the possible theoretical underpinnings of VR, drawing upon related psychological theories and frameworks that support its effectiveness as a therapeutic intervention.

DOI: 10.4324/9781003518327-6

4 Introduction to Virtual Reality

Introduction

Our previous section explored the principles of palliative care, traditional psychological interventions, and the unmet needs of patients in this critical context. This section proceeds to introduce VR interventions as an innovative approach with the potential to bridge the service gaps in existing palliative care practices. The current chapter begins by explaining the fundamentals of VR technology, focusing on its core principles of presence and immersion. It then celebrates the significant advancements in VR technology that emerge as an evidence-based therapeutic tool for treating various mental health conditions. The chapter also outlines the key advantages of using VR in mental health interventions, demonstrating how this innovative approach effectively addresses the shortcomings of conventional psychological methods. Moreover, with this advanced technology at our fingertips, we can bring hope and enhanced support to patients with terminal illnesses, paving the way for a more fulfilling end-of-life experience.

Virtual Reality

VR is defined as a three-dimensional (3D) virtual environment created by a computer that aims to reproduce a real environment or generate an imaginary world (Abbas et al., 2023). VR refers to an interface that connects the computer with human perceptual and/or muscle systems (Latta & Oberg, 1994). To establish a real-time relationship between the VR user and the virtual environment, a device is required to align the virtual content with the user's motion or intention (Mérienne, 2017). A head-tracking device, known as a head-mounted display, enables changes in the virtual environment to synchronize with the user's head movements such that the viewing experience resembles the real world (Wu et al., 2019). Such a device consists of input and output components. Motion tracking technology, as the input, is used to capture the user's physical motion and inform the computer to

DOI: 10.4324/9781003518327-7

adjust the virtual environment accordingly (Rolland & Hua, 2005). As the output, a visualization device with screen characteristics adjusted for close viewing is used to produce images (Mérienne, 2017).

The development of VR can be dated back to the 1960s when Ivan Sutherland created the first VR head-mounted display system (Werner, 2024). Early VR technology was primarily used for training in aviation and the military. At that time, VR devices were heavy, and computers lacked processing power (Rebenitsch, 2015). In the 1980s, the term "virtual reality" was coined by Jaron Lanier to represent a computer workstation with stereoscopic display, hand and gesture tracking, and 3D sound rendering (Bryson, 2013). In the 1990s, the mass production of VR emerged and reached a wider audience, and both commercial companies and researchers invested more resources into expanding the uses of VR (Gutiérrez et al., 2023). In the twenty-first century, VR has become readily accessible to the public and has significant untapped potential to be unleashed.

VR has been widely applied across different fields. One of the most popular current applications of VR is gaming, which leverages the engaging and enjoyable experience that VR can bring (Shelstad et al., 2017). Another application is in education and training. VR can provide practical training to reduce the costs and risks involved in creating a similar setting in real life—for example, for flight simulation, firefighting, and military operations (LaValle, 2023). In the healthcare industry, VR can be used by medical doctors to study the patient's 3D body before medical operations, explain medical options, or even directly deliver psychotherapies (Hsieh & Lee, 2017). During the COVID-19 outbreak, VR applications were an effective tool for supporting mental health (Pallavicini et al., 2021; Martirosov et al., 2022).

Virtual Reality and Presence

One distinctive feature of VR technology is the subjective sense of presence, which contributes to an authentic and immersive experience (Biocca, 1997). *Presence* refers to the psychological state of VR users, in which they perceive virtual experiences as being realistic (McCreery et al., 2013). Minsky (1980) was the first to use the concept of presence in the context of VR. Minsky characterized presence as a way for VR users to indirectly experience the world as if the VR user has been "transported" to another environment. Such an environment can be based on a real space (e.g., scenery captured by the camera) or an animated space generated by a computer (e.g., a non-existent world displayed in a video game) (Chalmers & Ferko, 2008).

Two major factors induce a sense of presence: vividness and interactivity (Steuer, 1995). *Vividness* refers to the sensory richness produced by the VR environment, which depends on sensory breadth (the number of senses presented at once) and sensory depth (the quality or clarity of the presented senses). On the other hand, *interactivity* refers to the extent to which VR users can affect the environment presented in the VR device, which depends on the time required for the user's input to be shown, the range of possible attributes the user can influence, and the number of changes the user can make.

For the VR environment to resemble reality, the social aspect of the users' experiences cannot be overlooked; these can be represented by social presence and co-presence. *Social presence* refers to the VR users' perceptions regarding the capacity of VR to establish a connection with others (Oh et al., 2018). When using VR while interacting with other people, social presence can offer extensive verbal and nonverbal information for interpersonal communication, as well as providing a sense of friendliness, warmth, sensitivity, and intimacy (Lombard & Ditton, 1997). *Co-presence* is related to the connection with other minds. Co-presence refers to the sense of "togetherness" among the parties involved, meaning that the VR user is actively perceiving others while others are also actively perceiving the VR user (Bulu, 2012). This mutual awareness places more emphasis on immediacy, affinity, and responsiveness to others (Pimentel & Vinkers, 2021). Such subjective feelings of connection with others appear to potentially address the unmet social needs of patients with terminal illnesses, who are limited by factors such as transportation barriers, poor physical health, and limited mobility (Fitzsimons et al., 2007), as discussed in Chapter 3.

Virtual Reality and Immersion

Immersion is another characteristic that is more prominent in VR than in other media forms. *Immersion* refers to the sense of being surrounded by something (Nilsson et al., 2016). Murray (1997) used the metaphor of "being submerged in water" to describe the experience of immersion, which feels as if our senses and attention are being taken over by stimuli in the virtual environment. Some researchers have used the term "immersion" interchangeably with the term "presence" (Nilsson et al., 2016). However, significant differences exist between the two concepts. Presence is a subjective perception that is influenced by VR content, whereas immersion encompasses the objective aspect of VR that is influenced by the technical quality of the VR system (Servotte et al., 2020). Mütterlein (2018) suggests that being present in the virtual environment or having few distractions from the real world is a prerequisite to being immersed in virtual activity.

Different levels of immersion depend on the extent of the user's isolation from the external environment, the user's perception of being included in the virtual environment, the use of natural actions for control, and the user's awareness of their movements (Witmer & Singer, 1998). Miller and Bugnariu (2016) identify three levels of immersion: low-immersive experiences are presented via a computer monitor without blocking the user's visual field, so users are prone to being affected by external disturbances; semi-immersive experiences make use of large-screen projection, with some elements in the virtual environment being available for interaction; and high-immersive experiences utilize devices that accommodate at least two sensory modalities, such as a head-mounted display or surround projection, thus creating a reality-like environment for users. When following these criteria for the three levels of immersion, VR can provide a highly immersive and fully engaging experience for users.

Immersion in VR has positive impacts on user performance. A meta-analysis by Coban and colleagues (2022) finds that teaching with immersive VR technologies is significantly more effective than teaching with other methods, such as computer-assisted teaching and traditional paper-and-pencil approaches. The effect of VR on user performance may increase with the level of immersion. Pollard and colleagues (2020) find that participants' spatial learning performance was significantly improved in a highly immersive condition than in a moderately immersive condition. These favourable results may be attributed to the ability of immersive VR to create a realistic and occlusive experience for users, which facilitates the efficient use of cognitive resources and enhances users' motivation via engaging media (Araiza-Alba et al., 2021; Pollard et al., 2020).

Immersion also brings positive health outcomes. De Zambotti et al. (2020) argue that VR has the potential to be a clinical tool to promote sleep, as it facilitates the falling asleep process in people with sleep-onset insomnia. Such sleep promotion can be achieved by distracting and immersing the user at bedtime in simulated relaxing realities that are designed to induce and control specific changes in mood and physiology that promote sleep-facilitating psychophysiological levels. A systematic review by Demeco and colleagues (2023) shows that the inclusion of fully immersive VR in the rehabilitation plan of stroke survivors helped improve their balance, gait performance, and limb dexterity. Furthermore, among patients with chronic neck pain undergoing fully immersive VR interventions, significantly greater improvements in subjective (e.g., self-reported pain intensity and disability) and objective measures (e.g., velocity and accuracy of neck movements) have been found, compared to groups receiving laser treatment or no treatment (Bahat et al., 2016). These advantages are made possible due to the immersive nature of VR, which directs the user's attention to training scenarios through the provision of alternative sensory inputs (Snoswell & Snoswell, 2019).

Virtual Reality and Mental Health

The use of VR has been associated with therapeutic benefits on mood and psychological well-being, which emerged as an alternative treatment tool for various mental disorders. Meta-analyses have revealed that VR-based exposure therapy is significantly effective in treating patients with social anxiety disorder (Horigome et al., 2020), post-traumatic stress disorder (Vianez et al., 2022), and obsessive-compulsive disorder (Dehghan et al., 2022). With a greater resemblance to real-life situations, the skills learned in VR-based interventions for psychosis are more generalizable, and treatment effects are more durable (Schroeder et al., 2022). The use of VR in patients with eating disorders has been found helpful for reducing body image disturbance (Cash & Grant, 1996), recognizing cognitive errors and changing eating habits (Riva, 2011), and reducing bulimia symptoms and dysfunctional behaviours (Roncero & Perpiñá, 2015). In targeting patients with substance-related disorders, exposing individuals to relevant drug cues through VR has been empirically studied to determine whether conditioned responses to substance use can be extinguished using VR (Culbertson et al., 2012; Kuntze et al., 2001). These promising results suggest that using VR to treat mental disorders will continue to be a growing avenue.

VR's potential for personalized experiences and adaptability to individual needs are characteristics that set it apart from conventional treatment approaches (du Plessis & Jordaan, 2024). Pardini and colleagues (2022) find that participants who were allowed to choose their preferred audio and visual elements for relaxation reported feeling more relaxed, immersed, and pleasant than those who had no choice options. Not all situations are suitable for patient self-adjustment, but this does not diminish the positive effects of VR treatment. Kritikos and colleagues (2021) tailor their VR-presented stimuli for use in exposure therapy for spider phobia according to the participant's immediate electrodermal activity and found higher treatment efficacy in the real-time adjustment group. Regardless of whether the treatment is adjusted in a client- or therapist-led manner, the personalization of VR interventions that are adapted to individual needs appears to enhance psychological well-being.

Besides its personalized nature, VR can bring positive affective impacts to its users via the presentation of a realistic natural environment. The exposure to a simulated natural environment brought by VR is known as virtual nature (Levi & Kocher, 1999); this overcomes the practical barriers, such as age, physical conditions, time, cost, and weather, that prevent people from visiting nature themselves (Yen et al., 2024). A systematic review by Frost and colleagues (2022) notes that immersion in a VR-created natural setting significantly reduces negative affect. Furthermore, Ma and colleagues (2023) find that VR-presented natural environments could facilitate mindfulness practice, resulting in higher positive mood and lower negative mood, showing the psychological benefits of virtual nature.

The psychological advantages of virtual nature may be explained by attention restoration theory (see Chapter 6 for more details), which posits that voluntary attention directed towards nature can activate the parasympathetic nervous system, thus fostering calmness and replenishing the attention required for daily tasks (Frost et al., 2022; Kaplan, 1995). A study by Gao and colleagues (2019) reports significantly lower negative mood and improved attention after participants view panoramic photographs of scenery via VR glasses. This shows that, with the immersive experience brought by the VR device and the resulting sense of presence, virtual nature can have similar benefits to being directly exposed to nature. Thus, this offers another direction for how VR can deliver positive affective impacts to its users.

In addition to the personalized and virtual nature of VR, VR has several other advantages over conventional treatment approaches. Rizzo and Bouchard (2019) report on the distinctive benefits of VR in anxiety treatment, which include but are not limited to the high degree of control that the therapist has over the anxiogenic object or situation, the cost-efficiency, and simplicity of VR relative to in vivo exposure, the use of VR as a flexible tool that allows replication of different physical environments, and VR as a viable alternative for individuals who consider that in vivo exposure is aversive.

Conclusions

This chapter lays the foundation for understanding the unique characteristics of VR, emphasizing concepts such as a sense of presence and immersion. It has traced the exciting advancements in VR technology that emerge as a promising therapeutic tool for various mental health conditions. The crossover of advanced technology and psychological methods appears to create unique opportunities for better outcomes in healthcare settings. The next chapter will introduce how VR has been studied in palliative care and is backed by both preliminary and robust research, illuminating pathways to improved experiences of patients at their end-of-life stage.

References

Abbas, J. R., O'Connor, A., Ganapathy, E., Isba, R., Payton, A., McGrath, B., Tolley, N., & Bruce, I. A. (2023). What is virtual reality? A healthcare-focused systematic review of definitions. *Health Policy and Technology, 12*(2), 100741. https://doi.org/10.1016/j.hlpt.2023.100741

Araiza-Alba, P., Keane, T., Chen, W. S., & Kaufman, J. (2021). Immersive virtual reality as a tool to learn problem-solving skills. *Computers and Education, 164,* 104121. https://doi.org/10.1016/j.compedu.2020.104121

Bahat, H. S., Croft, K., Hoddinott, A., Carter, C., & Treleaven, J. (2016). Remote kinematic e-training for patients with chronic neck pain, a randomised controlled trial. *Manual Therapy, 25,* e35. https://doi.org/10.1016/j.math.2016.05.030

Biocca, F. (1997). The cyborg's dilemma: Progressive embodiment in virtual environments [1]. *Journal of Computer-Mediated Communication*, *3*(2), 0. https://doi.org/10.1111/j.1083-6101.1997.tb00070.x

Bryson, S. (2013). Virtual reality: A definition history—a personal essay. *arXiv.org*. https://doi.org/10.48550/arxiv.1312.4322

Bulu, S. T. (2012). Place presence, social presence, co-presence, and satisfaction in virtual worlds. *Computers and Education*, *58*(1), 154–161. https://doi.org/10.1016/j.compedu.2011.08.024

Cash, T. F., & Grant, J. R. (1996). Cognitive-behavioral treatment of body image disturbances. In V. B. Van Hasselt & M. Hersen (Eds.), *Sourcebook of psychological treatment manuals for adult disorders*. Plenum Press.

Chalmers, A., & Ferko, A. (2008). Levels of realism: From virtual reality to real virtuality. In *Proceedings of the 24th spring conference on computer graphics* (pp. 19–25). https://doi.org/10.1145/1921264.1921272

Coban, M., Bolat, Y. I., & Goksu, I. (2022). The potential of immersive virtual reality to enhance learning: A meta-analysis. *Educational Research Review*, *36*, 100452. https://doi.org/10.1016/j.edurev.2022.100452

Culbertson, C. S., Shulenberger, S., De La Garza, R., Newton, T. F., Brody, A. L. (2012). Virtual reality cue exposure therapy for the treatment of tobacco dependence. *Journal of Cybertherapy and Rehabilitation*, *5*(1), 57–64.

de Zambotti, M., Barresi, G., Colrain, I. M., & Baker, F. C. (2020). When sleep goes virtual: The potential of using virtual reality at bedtime to facilitate sleep. *Sleep (New York, N.Y.)*, *43*(12), 1. https://doi.org/10.1093/sleep/zsaa178

Dehghan, B., Saeidimehr, S., Sayyah, M., & Rahim, F. (2022). The effect of virtual reality on emotional response and symptoms provocation in patients with OCD: A systematic review and meta-analysis. *Frontiers in Psychiatry*, *12*, 733584. https://doi.org/10.3389/fpsyt.2021.733584

Demeco, A., Zola, L., Frizziero, A., Martini, C., Palumbo, A., Foresti, R., Buccino, G., & Costantino, C. (2023). Immersive virtual reality in post-stroke rehabilitation: A systematic review. *Sensors (Basel, Switzerland)*, *23*(3), 1712. https://doi.org/10.3390/s23031712

du Plessis, J., & Jordaan, J. (2024). The impact of virtual reality on the psychological well-being of hospitalised patients: A critical review. *Heliyon*, *10*(2), e24831. https://doi.org/10.1016/j.heliyon.2024.e24831

Fitzsimons, D., Mullan, D., Wilson, J. S., Conway, B., Corcoran, B., Dempster, M., Gamble, J., Stewart, C., Rafferty, S., McMahon, M., MacMahon, J., Mulholland, P., Stockdale, P., Chew, E., Hanna, L., Brown, J., Ferguson, G., & Fogarty, D. (2007). The challenge of patients' unmet palliative care needs in the final stages of chronic illness. *Palliative Medicine*, *21*(4), 313–322. https://doi.org/10.1177/0269216307077711

Frost, S., Kannis-Dymand, L., Schaffer, V., Millear, P., Allen, A., Stallman, H., Mason, J., Wood, A., & Atkinson-Nolte, J. (2022). Virtual immersion in nature and psychological well-being: A systematic literature review. *Journal of Environmental Psychology*, *80*, 101765. https://doi.org/10.1016/j.jenvp.2022.101765

Gao, T., Zhang, T., Zhu, L., Gao, Y., & Qiu, L. (2019). Exploring psychophysiological restoration and individual preference in the different environments based on virtual reality. *International Journal of Environmental Research and Public Health*, *16*(17), 3102. https://doi.org/10.3390/ijerph16173102

Gutiérrez, M., Vexo, F., & Thalmann, D. (2023). Introduction. In *Stepping into virtual reality* (pp. 1–12). Springer. https://doi.org/10.1007/978-3-031-36487-7

Horigome, T., Kurokawa, S., Sawada, K., Kudo, S., Shiga, K., Mimura, M., & Kishimoto, T. (2020). Virtual reality exposure therapy for social anxiety disorder: A systematic review and meta-analysis. *Psychological Medicine, 50*(15), 2487–2497. https://doi.org/10.1017/S0033291720003785

Hsieh, M., & Lee, J. (2017). Preliminary study of VR and AR applications in medical and healthcare education. *Journal of Nursing and Health Studies, 3*(1), 1–5.

Kaplan, S. (1995). The restorative benefits of nature: Toward an integrative framework. *Journal of Environmental Psychology, 15*(3), 169–182. https://doi.org/10.1016/0272-4944(95)90001-2

Kritikos, J., Alevizopoulos, G., & Koutsouris, D. (2021). Personalized virtual reality human-computer interaction for psychiatric and neurological illnesses: A dynamically adaptive virtual reality environment that changes according to real-time feedback from electrophysiological signal responses. *Frontiers in Human Neuroscience, 15*, 596980. https://doi.org/10.3389/fnhum.2021.596980

Kuntze, M. F., Stoermer, R., Mager, R., Roessler, A., Mueller-Spahn, F., & Bullinger, A. H. (2001). Immersive virtual environments in cue exposure. *Cyberpsychology & Behavior, 4*(4), 497–501. https://doi.org/10.1089/109493101750527051

Latta, J. N., & Oberg, D. J. (1994). A conceptual virtual reality model. In *IEEE computer graphics and applications* (Vol. 14, No. 1, pp. 23–29). IEEE. https://doi.org/10.1109/38.250915

LaValle, S. M. (2023). Introduction. In *Virtual reality* (pp. 1–35). Cambridge University Press.

Levi, D., & Kocher, S. (1999). Virtual nature: The future effects of information technology on our relationship to nature. *Environment and Behavior, 31*(2), 203–226. https://doi.org/10.1177/00139169921972065

Lombard, M., & Ditton, T. (1997). At the heart of it all: The concept of presence. *Journal of Computer-Mediated Communication, 3*(2), 0. https://doi.org/10.1111/j.1083-6101.1997.tb00072.x

Ma, J., Zhao, D., Xu, N., & Yang, J. (2023). The effectiveness of immersive virtual reality (VR) based mindfulness training on improvement mental-health in adults: A narrative systematic review. *Explore (New York, N.Y.), 19*(3), 310–318. https://doi.org/10.1016/j.explore.2022.08.001

Martirosov, S., Bureš, M., & Zítka, T. (2022). Cyber sickness in low-immersive, semi-immersive, and fully immersive virtual reality. *Virtual Reality: The Journal of the Virtual Reality Society, 26*(1), 15–32. https://doi.org/10.1007/s10055-021-00507-4

McCreery, M. P., Schrader, P. G., Krach, S. K., & Boone, R. (2013). A sense of self: The role of presence in virtual environments. *Computers in Human Behavior, 29*(4), 1635–1640. https://doi.org/10.1016/j.chb.2013.02.002

Mérienne, F. (2017). Virtual reality: Principles and applications. In *Encyclopedia of computer science and technology* (pp. 1–11). Taylor and Francis. ff10.1081/E-ECST2-140000194ff.ffhal-01728062

Miller, H. L., & Bugnariu, N. L. (2016). Level of immersion in virtual environments impacts the ability to assess and teach social skills in autism spectrum disorder. *Cyberpsychology, Behavior and Social Networking, 19*(4), 246–256. https://doi.org/10.1089/cyber.2014.0682

Minsky, M. (1980). Telepresence. *OMNI Magazine*, 44–52. https://philpapers.org/rec/MINT

Murray, J. B. (1997). Immersion. In *Hamlet on the holodeck: The future of narrative in cyberspace* (pp. 95–125). Free Press.

Mütterlein, J. (2018). *The three pillars of virtual reality? Investigating the roles of immersion, presence, and interactivity.* Hawaii International Conference on System Sciences, Hawaii, United States. https://www.semanticscholar.org/paper/The-Three-Pillars-of-Virtual-Reality-Investigating-M%C3%BCtterlein/c0f6e6743d5d7c2caa9a8eb19ab7e604fbe3212d

Nilsson, N. C., Nordahl, R., & Serafin, S. (2016). Immersion revisited: A review of existing definitions of immersion and their relation to different theories of presence. *Human Technology*, *12*(2), 108–134. https://doi.org/10.17011/ht/urn.201611174652

Oh, C. S., Bailenson, J. N., & Welch, G. F. (2018). A systematic review of social presence: Definition, antecedents, and implications. *Frontiers in Robotics and AI*, *5*, 114. https://doi.org/10.3389/frobt.2018.00114

Pallavicini, F., Chicchi Giglioli, I. A., Kim, G. J., Alcañiz, M., & Rizzo, A. (2021). Editorial: Virtual reality, augmented reality and video games for addressing the impact of covid-19 on mental health. *Frontiers in Virtual Reality*, *2*. https://doi.org/10.3389/frvir.2021.719358

Pardini, S., Gabrielli, S., Dianti, M., Novara, C., Zucco, G., Mich, O., & Forti, S. (2022). The role of personalization in the user experience, preferences and engagement with virtual reality environments for relaxation. *International Journal of Environmental Research and Public Health*, *19*(12), 7237. https://doi.org/10.3390/ijerph19127237

Pimentel, D., & Vinkers, C. (2021). Copresence with virtual humans in mixed reality: The impact of contextual responsiveness on social perceptions. *Frontiers in Robotics and AI*, *8*, 634520. https://doi.org/10.3389/frobt.2021.634520

Pollard, K. A., Oiknine, A. H., Files, B. T., Sinatra, A. M., Patton, D., Ericson, M., Thomas, J., & Khooshabeh, P. (2020). Level of immersion affects spatial learning in virtual environments: Results of a three-condition within-subjects study with long intersession intervals. *Virtual Reality : The Journal of the Virtual Reality Society*, *24*(4), 783–796. https://doi.org/10.1007/s10055-019-00411-y

Rebenitsch, L. (2015). Managing cybersickness in virtual reality. *Crossroads (Association for Computing Machinery)*, *22*(1), 46–51. https://doi.org/10.1145/2810054

Riva, G. (2011). The key to unlocking the virtual body: Virtual reality in the treatment of obesity and eating disorders. *Journal of Diabetes Science and Technology*, *5*(2), 283–292. https://doi.org/10.1177/193229681100500213

Rizzo, A., & Bouchard, S. (2019). *Virtual reality for psychological and neurocognitive interventions.* Springer.

Rolland, J. P., & Hua, H. (2005). Head-mounted display systems. *Encyclopedia of Optical Engineering*, *2*, 1–14.

Roncero, M., & Perpiñá, C. (2015). Normalizing the eating pattern with virtual reality for bulimia nervosa: A case report. *Revista Mexicana de Trastornos Alimentarios*, *6*, 152–159. https://doi.org/10.1016/j.rmta.2015.11.001

Schroeder, A. H., Bogie, B. J. M., Rahman, T. T., Thérond, A., Matheson, H., & Guimond, S. (2022). Feasibility and efficacy of virtual reality interventions to improve psychosocial functioning in psychosis: Systematic review. *JMIR Mental Health*, *9*(2), e28502. https://doi.org/10.2196/28502

Servotte, J.-C., Goosse, M., Campbell, S. H., Dardenne, N., Pilote, B., Simoneau, I. L., Guillaume, M., Bragard, I., & Ghuysen, A. (2020). Virtual reality experience: Immersion, sense of presence, and cybersickness. *Clinical Simulation in Nursing*, *38*, 35–43. https://doi.org/10.1016/j.ecns.2019.09.006

Shelstad, W. J., Smith, D. C., & Chaparro, B. S. (2017). Gaming on the rift: How virtual reality affects game user satisfaction. *Proceedings of the Human Factors and Ergonomics Society Annual Meeting*, *61*(1), 2072–2076. https://doi.org/10.1177/1541931213602001

Snoswell, A. J., & Snoswell, C. L. (2019). Immersive virtual reality in health care: Systematic review of technology and disease states. *JMIR Biomedical Engineering*, *4*(1), e15025.

Steuer, J. (1995). Defining virtual reality: Dimensions determining telepresence. In F. Biocca & M. R. Levy (Eds.), *Communication in the age of virtual reality* (pp. 33–56). Lawrence Erlbaum Associates, Publishers.

Vianez, A., Marques, A., & Simões de Almeida, R. (2022). Virtual reality exposure therapy for armed forces veterans with post-traumatic stress disorder: A systematic review and focus group. *International Journal of Environmental Research and Public Health*, *19*(1), 464. https://doi.org/10.3390/ijerph19010464

Werner, J. (2024, February 23). Catchup with Ivan Sutherland—inventor of the first AR headset. *Forbes*. https://www.forbes.com/sites/johnwerner/2024/02/23/catchup-with-ivan-sutherlandinventor-of-the-first-ar-headset/

Witmer, B. G., & Singer, M. J. (1998). Measuring presence in virtual environments: A presence questionnaire. *Presence*, *7*(3), 225–240.

Wu, T. L. Y., Gomes, A., Fernandes, K., & Wang, D. (2019). The effect of head tracking on the degree of presence in virtual reality. *International Journal of Human-Computer Interaction*, *35*(17), 1569–1577. https://doi.org/10.1080/10447318.2018.1555736

Yen, H.-Y., Hsu, H., & Huang, W.-H. (2024). Virtual reality natural experiences for mental health: Comparing the effects between different immersion levels. *Virtual Reality: The Journal of the Virtual Reality Society*, *28*(1), 52. https://doi.org/10.1007/s10055-024-00958-5

5 Virtual Reality and Palliative Care

Introduction

"You matter because you are you, and you matter to the last moment of your life.
"We will do all we can not only to help you die peacefully, but also to live until you die."

(Saunders, 1967)

Cicely Saunders' poignant words highlight the inherent value of each patient throughout their life journey and the dedication of palliative care providers to ensure that patients can live fully until their final moments. At the heart of this mission lies the commitment to exploring diverse approaches that can maximize patient support. One example is the innovative application of VR technology, which has emerged as a transformative tool in palliative care, enabling what once seemed impossible. Emerging reviews and meta-analyses have been providing evidence to support its efficacy in symptom management. This chapter first introduces the scientific findings from these reviews, paving the way for a discussion that demonstrates how VR can specifically address patients' physical, psychological, social, and spiritual needs. The chapter then explores the application of VR in advance care planning, bereavement support, training and education, and psychological support for palliative care providers. It aims to showcase the global research and clinical efforts dedicated to maximizing the therapeutic use of VR in palliative care and establishing VR-assisted interventions as evidence-based practices that can significantly enhance the quality of end-of-life care.

Virtual Reality and Palliative Care

Systematic reviews have consistently pointed to the therapeutic potential of VR interventions in palliative care, suggesting that VR interventions are usable, feasible, and acceptable with promising outcomes in symptom management (Martin et al., 2022; Mo et al., 2022; Moloney et al., 2023; Moutogiannis et al., 2023). Specifically, Vasudevan et al. (2023) show that

DOI: 10.4324/9781003518327-8

using VR with patients receiving palliative care in a variety of settings results in positive outcomes and data on useability, feasibility, and acceptability. Huang et al. (2024) conduct a meta-synthesis of qualitative studies to explore the experiences and perceptions of palliative care patients undergoing VR therapy. The review identifies key themes, including patient experiences with VR, perceived benefits, and preferences for personalized therapy, highlighting the therapeutic potential of VR. Carmont and McIlfatrick (2022) identify VR's capacity to support not only patients but also families and healthcare professionals in the palliative care context. Please refer to Table 5.1 for details of the reviews and meta-analyses.

Virtual Reality Interventions Addressing Biopsychosocial–Spiritual Needs

Following an overview of the scientific evidence for VR interventions in palliative care settings, this section explores the uses of VR in addressing the specific needs of patients, particularly the unmet needs described in Chapter 3. The current section discusses how VR can facilitate adaptive coping in specific tasks that address patients' physical, psychological, social, and spiritual needs.

Physical Needs

Pain management is one of the most significant physical needs for patients with terminal illnesses (Deeken, 2004). Despite pharmaceutical interventions, unresolved pain remains an unmet need, as delineated in Chapter 3. Effective pain control has been impeded by both practical (Anekar et al., 2023) and patient-related obstacles (Jacobsen & colleagues, 2009). VR, as an alternative therapeutic tool, appears to bring some hope for suboptimal pain management. Emergent pilot studies have demonstrated the therapeutic potential of VR for pain control in patients under palliative care (Austin et al., 2022; Guenther et al., 2022; Johnson et al., 2020; Kelleher et al., 2022; Niki et al., 2019). For example, Laffer et al. (2023) present a feasible and clinically beneficial VR programme to improve pain and mood for veterans enrolled in hospice and palliative care. Burridge et al. (2023) evaluate the effectiveness of VR in reducing pain and anxiety for patients under palliative care in an acute hospital setting, presenting positive patient feedback on the VR experience. Randomized controlled trials have been conducted on pain management among patients with advanced heart failure (Groninger et al., 2021) and breast cancers (Mohammad & Ahmad, 2019); both trials support VR as an effective and safe nonpharmacologic adjuvant pain management intervention. Finally, Hartshorn et al. (2022) outline a protocol for a randomized controlled trial that assesses the efficacy of virtual

Table 5.1 Reviews and meta-analysis on the use of virtual reality in palliative care

First Author	Aim	Method	Results	Conclusions
Carmont and McIlfatrick (2022)	To review and synthesize evidence regarding the experiences of patients, families, and healthcare professionals in palliative care who have engaged with immersive/non-immersive VR technology.	A systematic integrative review using pre-defined MeSH search terms to identify eligible studies from five electronic databases (Cochrane Library, CINAHL, OVID Medline, Pubmed, and Scopus) between April 2020 and February 2021.	Rigorous analysis of eligible articles resulted in the identification of five overarching and interconnected themes: connection, VR as an emergent technology, perceptual change, safety, and future research.	This review identified that VR could support patients, families and healthcare professionals in palliative care. As a result of the COVID-19 pandemic, the findings could prove particularly significant for facilitating connection. However, further research is necessary to explore the full scope of VR use in this specialty.
Huang et al. (2024)	To explore the experiences and perceptions of patients receiving VR therapy in palliative care.	Ten databases, namely, PubMed, Web of Science, EBSCO, OVID MEDLINE, Scopus, John Wiley, ProQuest, CNKI, WANFANG DATA, and SinoMed, were searched, and qualitative and mixed studies from the establishment of each database to June 30, 2023, were included.	Three key themes were identified: experiences of palliative care patients in VR therapy, the perceived value that palliative care patients gain in VR therapy, and perspectives of palliative care patients toward using VR therapy.	The findings indicated that VR therapy may be an effective approach to relieve patients' physical and psychological pain and help them gain self-awareness.
Martin et al. (2022)	To synthesize the available research on the use of VR for enhancing psychological and somatic outcomes for palliative care patients. Secondary aims included assessing general satisfaction and overall usability.	A pre-registered systematic literature search according to PRISMA guidelines using OVID Emcare, Cochrane Library, Embase, Medline, PsycINFO, and PubMed Care Search: Palliative Care Knowledge Network, between 2019 and 2021.	While the reported quantitative psychological and somatic outcomes were ambiguous, the qualitative outcomes were largely positive. Participants were generally satisfied with VR, and most studies reported the VR interventions as usable, feasible, and acceptable.	VR shows promise in palliative care and generally addresses a range of symptoms with few adverse effects. Future research should consist of adequately powered RCTs evaluating dosage and focusing on providing meaningful activities to enhance outcomes further.

(Continued)

Table 5.1 (Continued)

First Author	Aim	Method	Results	Conclusions
Mo et al. (2022)	To determine the feasibility and effectiveness of virtual reality use within a palliative care setting.	Data sources: Medline, Embase, AMED, PsycINFO, CINAHL, Cochrane Central Register of Controlled Trials, and Web of Science were searched from inception to March 2021. Search terms included "virtual reality" and "palliative care."	VR statistically significantly improved pain (p = 0.0363), tiredness (p = 0.0030), drowsiness (p = 0.0051), shortness of breath (p = 0.0284), depression (p = 0.0091) and psychological well-being (p = 0.0201). The quality of the evidence was graded as very low due to small sample sizes, non-randomization methods and a lack of a comparator arm.	Virtual reality in palliative care is feasible and acceptable. However, limited sample sizes and very low-quality studies mean that the efficacy of virtual reality needs further research.
Moloney et al. (2023)	To chart the literature on virtual reality use in palliative care, identifying any evidence relating to biopsychosocial patient outcomes which could support its use in practice.	A scoping review of the literature involving a systematic search across 10 electronic bibliographic databases in December 2021. Eligibility criteria were primary research studies of any research design within a 10-year timeframe, which reported on virtual reality use and patient outcomes in palliative care.	VR use with patients receiving palliative care in a variety of settings, and data around useability, feasibility, and acceptability is positive. However, the evidence regarding biopsychosocial patient outcomes linked to virtual reality use is limited.	Virtual reality is gathering momentum in palliative care and is potentially a helpful intervention; however, more research is needed to underpin the evidence base supporting its application, particularly in understanding the impact on biopsychosocial patient outcomes and ascertaining the best approach for measuring intervention effectiveness.

(*Continued*)

Table 5.1 (Continued)

First Author	Aim	Method	Results	Conclusions
Moutogiannis et al. (2023)	To present the current literature on the uses and benefits of VR for palliative care and hospice patients.	A systematic review involving 14 articles published between 2018 and 2023 that used VR as an interventional strategy for symptom management.	Virtual reality software was contained exclusively in the head-mounted displays or required a laptop. Nature scenes, memorable locations, and the solar system are examples of options patients could select for the VR experience. Assessments of the intervention were measured before, during, after, and several hours afterward to evaluate benefits and potential adverse effects. Pain was the predominant symptom assessed in the studies.	Most of the studies focused on establishing the safety, efficacy, and feasibility of VR using a single-arm interventional method. Future research should implement randomized controlled trials, increase sample size, and expand to paediatric populations.
Vasudevan et al. (2023)	To understand design trends, gaps, and opportunities for VR in palliative care.	A literature search conducted in April 2023 using four databases: Scopus, Association for Computing Machinery (ACM), Institute of Electronic Engineers (IEEE Xplore), and PsycINFO.	The design and use of VR in the PC setting demonstrating aspects of palliative care that VR currently supports: symptom management, embedded enrichment, personalized care, and decision-making, with the former dominating the field. Dominant design strategies included: active vs. passive engagement in VR, narrative building, and supporting accessibility and mobility. Participatory approaches were underutilized. VR currently takes an interventionist approach, focusing on clinical outcomes.	Current VR experiences have shown great promise in supporting aspects of a holistic model of care in adult PC populations.

reality-assisted guided imagery (VRAGI) for pain management in patients with advanced cancer in a home setting.

VR interventions do not only assist in pain management, but they also address various other physical symptoms. In a prospective study of 30 patients in a regional hospice, a 15-minute video of serene nature scenes with ambient sounds is found to significantly improve total symptom scores, as well as scores for drowsiness, tiredness, depression, anxiety, well-being, and dyspnoea (Deming et al., 2024). Moon et al. (2023) investigate the "Godrevy Project," which utilizes VR for symptom control and well-being in oncology and patients under palliative care. The researchers conclude that VR is an effective, patient-controlled, nonpharmacological intervention without significant side effects. Similarly, VR is considered to be a potential therapeutic tool for total rehabilitation (Filho et al., 2022).

The personalized nature of VR content appears to be associated with the management of physical symptoms. Altman et al. (2024) evaluate the role of personalized VR in palliative care, focusing on its effects on symptom management and quality of life for patients, with their findings suggesting clinically meaningful improvements. A randomized controlled trial conducted by Woo et al. (2024) reports how a personalized VR psychological intervention outperformed traditional relaxation therapy, with a greater reduction in physical and psychological symptoms in the VR group. The feasibility trial of Perna et al. (2021) advocates the potential of personalized VR in palliative care. Finally, Gerlach et al. (2023) present a mixed-methods study protocol focusing on the needs of patients in palliative cancer care using individualized VR content. Their approach aims to assess how customized VR experiences can impact patient care and emotional support. Please refer to Table 5.2 for various studies on the management of physical symptoms.

Among children or adolescents with terminal illnesses, a case report from Weingarten et al. (2020) advocates the endless potential of VR interventions in paediatric palliative care, while an exploratory trial (Wong et al., 2022) has demonstrated the potential effectiveness, feasibility, and acceptability of immersive VR for managing anxiety and acute nausea amongst paediatric patients with cancer receiving their first chemotherapy. The results of another randomized controlled trial conducted by Wong et al. (2021) indicate that VR is safe and effective for alleviating pain and anxiety among paediatric cancer patients undergoing peripheral intravenous cannulation procedures. Please refer to Table 5.3 for various studies on symptom management in paediatric palliative care.

Based on homecare settings, a brief research report by Moscato et al. (2021) supports the idea that VR could be a suitable complementary tool for the treatment of pain and mood in advanced cancer patients who are assisted at home. A randomized controlled trial by Maddox et al. (2023) finds that an eight-week self-administered in-home VR programme produces

Table 5.2 Management of physical symptoms

First Author	Research Title	Aim	VR Content
Altman et al. (2024)	Personalized virtual reality in palliative care: clinically meaningful symptom improvement for some.	To evaluate VR therapy benefits across three sessions, assessing its differential impact on emotional versus physical symptoms and determining the proportion of patients experiencing clinically meaningful improvements after each session.	Three personalized 20 minute VR sessions
Austin et al. (2022)	Feasibility and acceptability of virtual reality for cancer pain in people receiving palliative care: a randomized cross-over study.	To determine the feasibility and preliminary effectiveness for larger randomized controlled trials of 3D head-mounted (HMD) virtual reality for managing cancer pain (CP) in adults.	3D head-mounted virtual reality for managing cancer pain (3D HMD VR)
Burridge et al. (2023)	Winner of the Marlow prize: Virtual reality reduced pain and anxiety for palliative care patients in an acute hospital setting: A service evaluation.	To evaluate the feasibility and outcomes of VR in palliative care, particularly in the acute hospital setting.	Approximately 7 minutes VR session
Corvin et al. (2024)	The effects of virtual reality interventions on occupational participation and distress from symptoms in palliative care patients: A pilot study.	To examine the effect of VR interventions on occupational participation and distress from symptoms.	One VR session lasting from 9 to 30 minutes related to coping with pain, inner peace and mindfulness, adventure, and bucket list
Deming et al. (2024)	Virtual Reality Videos for Symptom Management in Hospice and Palliative Care.	To learn more about the effect of VR videos on patients' symptoms near the end of life, including which are most effective, how long the effect lasts, and which patients benefit the most.	15-minute video of serene nature scenes with ambient sounds

(Continued)

Table 5.2 (Continued)

First Author	Research Title	Aim	VR Content
Filho et al. (2022)	Immersive virtual reality in palliative care: prospects for total rehabilitation.	To discuss the promising role of immersive virtual reality in palliative care rehabilitation and propose the concept of total rehabilitation as a possibility to expand the current conception of rehabilitation.	-
Gerlach et al. (2023)	My virtual home: needs of patients in palliative cancer care and content effects of individualized virtual reality—a mixed methods study protocol.	To assess if VR videos with content tailored to the individual palliative cancer in patient's desire to be at home is accepted and suitable to improve their quality of life.	VR videos of their choice (their home, relatives, others if applicable)
Groninger et al. (2021)	Virtual reality for pain management in advanced heart failure: a randomized controlled study.	To investigate the impact of a virtual reality experience on self-reported pain, quality-of-life, general distress, and satisfaction compared to a two-dimensional guided imagery active control.	Virtual reality session with 10-minute guide through a forest and waterfall with voice narration
Guenther et al. (2022)	Virtual reality reduces pain in palliative care–A feasibility trial.	To investigate the feasibility of a single VR experience as a viable, satisfying, and effective tool for end-of-life pain relief for inpatients presenting palliative needs.	360° videos or games for relaxation, distraction, or escaping reality
Hartshorn et al. (2022)	Efficacy of virtual reality assisted guided imagery (VRAGI) in a home setting for pain management in patients with advanced cancer: protocol for a randomized controlled trial.	To test the impact of Virtual Reality Assisted Guided Imagery (VRAGI) as a complementary treatment modality to manage chronic pain in patients with cancer on patients with advanced cancer in a home setting.	Virtual Reality Assisted Guided Imagery (VRAGI)

(Continued)

Table 5.2 (Continued)

First Author	Research Title	Aim	VR Content
Johnson et al. (2020)	Virtual reality use for symptom management in palliative care: a pilot study to assess user perceptions.	To examine the utility of VR for palliative care patients.	Photorealistic images of popular real-world destinations and landscapes combined with audio/animated videos/simulations of rocket launches and space travel (Apollo 11 and Hello Mars)/simulation of a roller coaster (Coaster)
Kelleher et al. (2022)	Virtual reality for improving pain and pain-related symptoms in patients with advanced stage colorectal cancer: A pilot trial to test feasibility and acceptability.	To examine the feasibility, acceptability, safety, and impact of a 30-minute virtual underwater/sea environment (VR Blue) for reducing pain and pain-related symptoms in advanced colorectal cancer patients.	Immersive virtual reality in a 30-minute virtual underwater/sea environment
Laffer et al. (2023)	Implementation of virtual reality to improve quality of life for veterans in hospice and palliative care.	To investigate and interdisciplinary VR program aimed at improving the quality of life for veterans receiving inpatient hospice and palliative care.	-
Lloyd and Haraldsdottir (2021)	Virtual reality in hospice: improved patient well-being.	To trial the technology and consider what benefits may emerge for hospice in patients.	30-minute virtual travel, participants selected the destination of their choice, session guided by a facilitator
Mohammad and Ahmad (2019)	Virtual reality as a distraction technique for pain and anxiety among patients with breast cancer: A randomized control trial.	To assess the effectiveness of immersive virtual reality (VR) distraction technology in reducing pain and anxiety among female patients with breast cancer.	Immersive virtual reality distraction technology, choosing from two scenarios: deep sea diving or sitting on a beach

(Continued)

Table 5.2 (Continued)

First Author	Research Title	Aim	VR Content
Moon et al.	"Godrevy Project": virtual reality for symptom control and well-being in oncology and palliative care—a non-randomized pre-post interventional trial.	To determine whether VR intervention brings along an effective improvement in symptom control and well-being.	Self-selection from 18 VR videos filmed in various locations around Cornwall, The Isles of Scilly, and Europe
Niki et al. (2019)	A novel palliative care approach using virtual reality for improving various symptoms of terminal cancer patients: a preliminary prospective, multicentre study.	To verify whether simulated travel using virtual reality (VR travel) is efficacious in improving symptoms in terminal cancer patients.	Simulated virtual reality travel to the destination according to participants' wishes
Woo and Lee (2023)	Case report: Therapeutic potential of Flourishing-Life-Of-Wish Virtual Reality Therapy on Relaxation (FLOW-VRT-Relaxation)— a novel personalized .relaxation in palliative care	To develop, and test the feasibility and usability of FLOW-VRT-Relaxation as a new protocol for its potential to personalized yet scalable and cost-effective.	YouTube VR
Woo et al. (2024)	Flourishing-Life-Of-Wish Virtual Reality Relaxation Therapy (FLOW-VRT-Relaxation) outperforms traditional relaxation therapy in palliative care: results from a randomized controlled trial.	To test the efficacy of FLOW-VRT-Relaxation in effective symptom control, i.e, improved emotional and physical symptoms, when compared with a traditional relaxation practice.	FLOW-VRT-Relaxation

Table 5.3 Symptom management in paediatric palliative care

First Author	Research Title	Aim	VR Content
Weingarten et al. (2020)	Virtual reality: endless potential in pediatric palliative care: a case report.	To investigate the feasibility, acceptability, and potential use of VR in paediatric palliative care.	Personalized 360° video offered by company "Wishplay"
Wong et al. (2021)	Virtual reality intervention targeting pain and anxiety among pediatric cancer patients undergoing peripheral intravenous cannulation: A randomized controlled trial.	To determine whether virtual reality distraction intervention can alleviate pain and anxiety and reduce the length of procedure among paediatric cancer patients undergoing.	VR app
Wong et al. (2022)	Effects of immersive virtual reality for managing anxiety, nausea and vomiting among paediatric cancer patients receiving their first chemotherapy: An exploratory randomized controlled trial.	To assess the feasibility and acceptability of immersive virtual reality for managing anxiety, nausea, and vomiting amongst paediatric patients with cancer receiving their first chemotherapy.	VR app

clinically meaningful improvements in pain intensity and interference in clinically severe and diverse adults with chronic low back pain. Hoffman et al. (2014) discuss a feasible, safe, well-tolerated, and highly acceptable home-based exercise intervention that targets fatigue in patients undergoing adjuvant treatment. Please refer to Table 5.4 for various studies on symptom management using VR in-home support.

Psychological Needs

The need for self-determination and taking an active role has been advocated in patients under palliative care (Deeken, 2004). This is similar to the sense of autonomy described by Houska and Loučka (2019) as "being normal" and "taking charge." "Being normal" involves perceiving the body as normal despite the physical changes resulting from illness symptoms, while "taking charge" refers to being able to control preparations for the end of life, such as being able to make decisions and fulfil one's own needs. As discussed in Chapter 3, patients in palliative care continue to experience unfulfilled autonomy needs. Capitalizing on the characteristics and opportunities of action and control (Gaggioli et al., 2003), VR appears to have

Table 5.4 In-home support

First Author	Research Title	Aim	VR Content
Moscato et al. (2021)	Virtual reality in-home palliative care: brief report on the effect on cancer-related symptomatology.	To assess the effect of an immersive VR-based intervention conducted at home on anxiety, depression, and pain over four days and to evaluate the short-term effect of VR sessions on cancer-related symptomatology.	Immersive VR-based intervention
Hoffman et al. (2014)	Virtual reality bringing a new reality to postthoracotomy lung cancer patients via a home-based exercise intervention targeting fatigue while undergoing adjuvant treatment.	To investigate the feasibility, acceptability, and preliminary efficacy of an exercise intervention for postthoracotomy NSCLC patients including those initiating and completing adjuvant therapy.	Home-based exercise intervention promoted light-intensity walking and balance exercises utilizing an efficacy-enhancing virtual-reality approach using the Nintendo Wii Fit Plus.
Maddox et al. (2023)	In-home virtual reality program for chronic lower back pain: a randomized sham-controlled effectiveness trial in a clinically severe and diverse sample.	To determine whether an 8-week, self-administered in-home, behavioural skills virtual reality program for chronic low back pain (RelieVRx) that trains diaphragmatic breathing, biofeedback, cognition and emotion regulation, mindfulness, and pain education skills, is superior to a strong active Sham at day 56 for improving pain intensity and pain interference, in a large real-world sample.	The app consists of multiple pain education, relaxation, biofeedback, mindfulness, and breathing modules. Supported by RCT with an adequate sample size and approved by US Food and Drug Administration.

a high potential to facilitate a sense of self-determination or autonomy by allowing patients to select any activities in the virtual world without the boundaries of place, time, and people. An article by Irving (2023) highlights how VR provides hospice patients with a special opportunity to fulfil long-held desires and create meaningful moments for patients in palliative care settings. A case report by Woo and Lee (2023) reports using VR to fulfil the psychological need of wish fulfilment through virtual travel to the dream place of a patient with terminal cancer. In a dementia hospice setting, Ferguson et al. (2020) endorses the acceptability, tolerability, and enjoyment of VR interventions as a new alternative for therapeutic recreation among patients.

There is supportive evidence for VR interventions that specifically target the emotional needs of patients with end-of-life challenges. A study by Baños et al. (2013) advocate the feasibility and possible benefits of a psychological intervention that uses VR to induce positive emotions in adult hospitalized patients with metastatic cancer. The researchers report adequate levels of pleasantness with the main perceived benefits of distraction, entertainment, and the promotion of relaxation states. Burridge et al. (2023) evaluate the feasibility of VR in reducing anxiety and pain for palliative care patients in an acute hospital setting, presenting positive patient feedback on the VR experience. Corvin et al. (2024) examine the impact of VR interventions on occupational participation and symptom distress in palliative care patients, reporting significant improvements in occupational performance and satisfaction, as well as decreases in pain and fatigue distress. Their pilot study highlights VR as a promising therapeutic modality in both community-based and inpatient palliative care settings. Lastly, Brungardt et al. (2021) find that most participants speak favourably of a VR-based music therapy intervention, describing pleasant emotional and physical responses. The research team, led by the same principal investigator, later explores the patient outcomes of a pilot programme implementing VR-based music therapy in palliative care; they find moderate clinical improvements in physical and emotional symptoms, as well as small improvements in quality of life (Brungardt et al., 2024). Please refer to Table 5.5 for various studies on the management of psychological symptoms using VR.

Social Needs

The need for companionship is especially crucial for patients with terminal illnesses (Deeken, 2004), yet social isolation and inadequate emotional support continue to be significant unmet needs in palliative care, as outlined in Chapter 3. Social isolation may be attributed to structural and community-level factors such as transportation barriers and patient-related factors such as mobility restrictions and feelings of embarrassment that are related to a lack of control over symptoms (Fitzsimons et al., 2007; Ritchie & Kotwal, 2023).

Capitalizing on the sense of social presence (Lombard & Ditton, 1997), VR appears to provide an alternative to overcoming obstacles through a sense of companionship in the virtual environment. Niki et al. (2024) newly investigate the use of real-time virtual outings through VR for hospitalized patients with mobility challenges and personal requests to communicate virtually with loved family members. The results show that the patients and their families could enjoy smooth conversations without time lags, which highlights the therapeutic potential of VR intervention to enhance patients' unmet social needs. In a study by Mukai et al. (2023), family members of patients in hospital-based palliative care are asked to take videos of themselves

Table 5.5 Psychological symptom management

First Author	Research Title	Aim	VR Content
Baños et al. (2013)	A positive psychological intervention using virtual reality for patients with advanced cancer in a hospital setting: a pilot study to assess feasibility.	To examine the feasibility and possible benefits of a psychological intervention that uses virtual reality to induce positive emotions on adult hospitalized patients with metastatic cancer.	Navigation through a virtual environment to induce joy and relaxation
Brungardt et al. (2021)	Virtual reality-based music therapy in palliative care: a pilot implementation trial.	To evaluate implementation measures of feasibility, usability, and acceptability of a VR-based music therapy intervention.	Virtual reality-based music therapy with customized soundtrack
Brungardt et al. (2024)	Patient Outcomes of a Virtual Reality-Based Music Therapy Pilot in Palliative Care.	To assess symptom distress and quality of life among hospitalized palliative care patients who participated in a virtual reality-based music therapy (VR-MT) intervention and to explore VR-MT from the perspectives of health care professionals involved in their care.	Virtual reality-based music therapy
Ferguson et al. (2020)	Virtual reality for therapeutic recreation in dementia hospice care: A feasibility study.	To explore acceptability, tolerability, and subjective experience of virtual reality (VR) as therapeutic recreation for hospice patients living with dementia.	Virtual Reality for therapeutic recreation
Mukai et al. (2023)	Virtual reality images of the home are useful for patients with hospital-based palliative care: prospective observational study with analysis by text mining.	To clarify the usefulness of VR viewing for this purpose by text mining interviews with the patients in palliative care after their VR experience and to clarify the feasibility of this program.	Personalized VR content of persons or places familiar to participants
Nwosu et al. (2024)	Virtual reality in specialist palliative care: a feasibility study to enable clinical practice adoption.	To explore the feasibility of implementing VR therapy for patients and caregivers in a hospital specialist inpatient palliative care unit and a hospice.	VR distraction therapy. Oculus Gear VR store downloads, including a 5-minute guided relaxation video of a beach, a 10-minute guided meditation through a computer-generated forest, a 5-minute video roller coaster ride
Perna et al (2021)	The potential of personalized virtual reality in palliative care: a feasibility trial.	To understand the feasibility of repeated personalized virtual reality sessions in a palliative care population.	Personalized virtual reality experience using VR video available online based on participants' preference

at home and other familiar places where the patients wished to visit using a 3D camera. The study results, which are attained by text mining, suggest that VR has promising potential for relieving the pain of hospitalization by helping patients to feel safe and secure through virtual contact with family members and providing an immersive feeling of being in the same space as them. Besides, a (project by...) A project by Mackey et al. (2020) aims to design and implement an immersive control system for a robotic surrogate that allows users to interact as naturally as possible with their loved ones from a remote location and navigate appropriately. Ando et al. (2020) develop a group peer support and exercise intervention in which an avatar is created in the virtual world with the virtual exercise trainer. Finally, Knowles et al. (2017) make use of online, real-time, interactive VR and online avatars to promote feelings of inclusion and help widowers process feelings of grief. Please refer to Table 5.6 for various studies on VR interventions for social support interventions.

Spiritual Needs

The need for life review is highlighted in patients under palliative care (Deeken, 2004). Reminiscence therapy, or life review interventions, are found effective in addressing the spiritual needs of patients with terminal illnesses (Ando et al., 2007; Deeken, 2004; Wang et al., 2017; Warth et al., 2019). Such interventions aim to improve self-esteem and facilitate a sense of fulfilment by helping patients review their past lives and discuss their past experiences (Park et al., 2019; O'Philbin et al., 2018). As a lack of meaning in life is an unmet need among patients with terminal illnesses, life review interventions may help foster a sense of purpose and significance in patients' lives.

As reminiscence therapy is normally prompted by memory cues or triggers such as photographs, music, or meaningful objects (Kiernat, 1979), VR appears to provide more vivid, realistic, and interactive memory triggers that smooth the reminiscence, thereby further improving the patient's mood or other palliative symptoms. A feasibility study by Dang et al. (2021) report on an avatar-facilitated life review using a synchronized personalized avatar in VR. This uses an avatar storytelling platform that includes five environments that could be selected by the patient (i.e., beach, mountain, city, living room, and empty space) and 64 customized avatar options (i.e., four male and four female avatars at each of four developmental stages: child, teenager, adult, and elder). Ryu and Price (2022) report the VoicingHan avatar life-review for embodied storytelling and meaning-making at the end of life in patients with cancer under palliative care. Another study by Ng et al. (2024) invites six clinical psychologists to experience and evaluate a newly developed VR life review therapy system, concluding that the system

Table 5.6 Social support intervention

First Author	Research Title	Aim	VR Content
Ando et al. (2020)	Tele Virtual Reality-based Peer Support Programme for Cancer Patients: A Preliminary Feasibility and Acceptability Study.	To examine the feasibility and acceptability of the Tele Virtual Reality-based Peer Support Programme for Cancer Patients.	Unity
Knowles et al. (2017)	A pilot study of virtual support for grief: Feasibility, acceptability, and preliminary outcomes. Computers in Human Behavior.	To examine the feasibility and acceptability of an online, real-time, interactive VR support group for widow(er)s and to assess the preliminary efficacy of the VR support group for improving psychosocial outcomes and sleep quality compared to an active control grief education website.	Second Life®
Mackey et al. (2020)	Immersive control of a robot surrogate for users in palliative care.	To design and implement an immersive control system for a robotic surrogate that allows users to interact as naturally as possible with their loved ones from a remote location and navigate appropriately in order to improve the quality of life for those living with a terminal illness.	Head-mounted display (HMD) based control system for a Pepper robot
Niki et al. (2024)	A real-time virtual outing using virtual reality for a hospitalized terminal cancer patient who has difficulty going out: a case report.	To explore the feasibility of implementing the real-time virtual outing.	A 360° video real-time sharing system to broadcast the view of the daughter's home.

is feasible and effective for use with patients under palliative care. Please refer to Table 5.7 for various studies on the use of VR in spiritual support interventions.

Virtual Reality Interventions Addressing Other Needs

In addition to supporting patients' individual needs, the application of VR has been studied in the field of advance care planning, bereavement support, training and education, and psychological support provision for palliative care providers.

Advance Care Planning

As described in Chapter 3, barriers exist that prevent proactive engagement in advance care planning (ACP), leaving it as an unmet need in palliative care. For instance, some patients in palliative care have limited awareness and relevant knowledge, while others find the concept of ACP abstract and challenging to comprehend (Kim & Flieger, 2023; Nagelschmidt et al., 2021). VR appears to provide an innovative and helpful tool to address this issue. Hsieh (2020) develops a six-minute VR video with a first-person perspective on a patient with chronic obstructive pulmonary disease to allow VR participants to immerse themselves in the complete clinical process of

Table 5.7 Spiritual support intervention

First Author	Research Title	Aim	VR Content
Dang et al. (2021)	Feasibility of delivering an avatar-facilitated life review intervention for patients with cancer.	To determine the feasibility of an avatar-based intervention for facilitating life review in patients with advanced cancer.	An avatar-facilitated life review
Ryu and Price (2022)	Embodied storytelling and meaning-making at the end of life: VoicingHan avatar life-review for palliative care in cancer patients.	To discuss the theoretical frameworks for life-review and assess the benefits of the VoicingHan avatar system.	An avatar-facilitated life review
Ng et al. (2024)	Participatory design of a virtual reality life review therapy system for palliative care.	To evaluate the novel virtual reality life review therapy system.	A therapy space in a typical *Tong Lau* building to encourage life reflection

typical end-of-life care. After viewing the VR video, the preference for not using cardiopulmonary resuscitation, life-sustaining treatment, and other medical interventions increases significantly in the VR intervention group compared with the participants in the control group, who only complete pre-test and post-test questionnaires. Uncertainty regarding the available medical options also significantly decreases.

Chang et al. (2024) assess the effectiveness of a VR teaching module on ACP for medical professionals, aiming to improve their knowledge and skills in handling end-of-life issues. They report that medical professionals have better knowledge of ACP, improved attitudes toward ACP, and greater confidence in implementing advance decisions after experiencing the VR module. The findings also suggest that a VR format may help motivate medical professionals to perform essential actions related to making advance decisions, including introducing advance decisions to their patients and discussing them with their own families. Please refer to Table 5.8 for an overview of studies on the use of VR for ACP.

Bereavement Support

By embracing a holistic approach, palliative care offers support not only to patients but also to their families and significant others. Some clinical units provide continual psychological services to address the anticipatory grief

Table 5.8 Advance Care Planning

First Author	Research Title	Aim	VR Content
Chang et al. (2024)	The effectiveness of a virtual reality teaching module on advance care planning and advance decision for medical professionals.	To evaluate the effectiveness of a virtual reality teaching module on advance care planning and advance decisions for medical professionals.	A VR teaching module to help medical professionals better understand advance care planning and advance directives/decisions, with assessment tools integrated into the module
Hsieh (2020)	Virtual reality video promotes effectiveness in advance care planning.	To explore the change in participants' preference and certainty regarding end-of-life decisions after using VR video that promotes effectiveness in advance care planning.	Virtual reality video for advanced care planning

and bereavement of family members. VR appears to play a role in supporting adjustment during bereavement. A case report by Botella et al. (2008) describes the design of a VR environment (EMMA's World) for fostering the expression and processing of emotions and provides preliminary support for its use in treating complicated grief. A pilot study conducted by Knowles et al. (2017) demonstrate the feasibility, acceptability, and preliminary efficacy of a low-cost, online, interactive, and real-time VR support group for widow(er)s. Quero et al. (2019) investigate an adaptive VR system for the treatment of adjustment disorder and complicated grief, with the results showing significant improvements in psychological symptoms. Liao et al. (2023) design a VR grief farewell scene that aims to assist bereaved children to bid farewell to their deceased relatives and regain their confidence in life.

In the face of feasibility and pilot studies in the field, Pizzoli et al. (2023) critically discuss the possible side effects of VR interventions, as well as the hypothetical therapeutical applications of VR for the treatment of mourning. They highlight the fact that VR involves content related to grief, which is a dramatic yet natural experience, and putting fragile subjects in virtual environments can have deep psychological impacts on the user. Further clinical and research studies are therefore essential to ensure the ethical use of VR among this vulnerable population in their mourning process. Please refer to Table 5.9 for various studies on the use of VR for bereavement support.

Training and Education

VR has also been applied in training healthcare professionals, particularly in enhancing their communication skills, multidisciplinary collaborations, and understanding of palliative care. In terms of training, Andrade et al. (2010) study the use of VR with avatar interaction to enhance the communication abilities of medical students breaking bad news. Tan et al. (2013) use interactive computer simulations of real-life clinical scenarios to train, educate, and assess health professionals. In a mixed-methods study, Zhang et al. (2024) examine the impact of virtual clinical simulations on nursing students' palliative care knowledge, skills, and attitudes, emphasizing the benefits of immersive training experiences. Hall et al. (2024) also investigate among the nursing students the effectiveness of simulated participants and VR simulations in enhancing communication skills in end-of-life care. To improve accessibility while maintaining the effectiveness of evidence-based training in emergency settings, a study that incorporates VR technology into palliative care communication training demonstrates that a streamlined 360-degree VR environment allows clinicians to practise essential communication skills in just one hour (Ouchi, 2023). To facilitate understanding of palliative care, Taubert et al. (2019) use immersive VR to enhance medical

Table 5.9 VR and bereavement support

First Author	Research Title	Aim	VR Content
Botella et al. (2008)	Treatment of Complicated Grief Using Virtual Reality: A Case Report.	To explore the application of new technologies, concretely virtual reality, to facilitate emotional processing in the treatment of Complicated Grief.	A self-designed virtual reality environment (EMMA's World)
Knowles et al. (2017)	A pilot study of virtual support for grief: Feasibility, acceptability, and preliminary outcomes.	To examine the feasibility and acceptability of an online, real-time, interactive virtual reality (VR) support group for widow(er)s, and assess the preliminary efficacy of the VR support group for improving psychosocial outcomes and sleep quality compared to an active control grief education website.	A VR support group
Liao et al. (2023)	A grief farewell scene design for children based on virtual reality.	To investigate the effectiveness of a newly-developed virtual reality grief farewell scene designed to help bereaved children bid farewell to their deceased relatives and regain their confidence in life.	A virtual reality grief farewell scene
Pizzoli et al. (2023)	From virtual to real healing: a critical overview of the therapeutic use of virtual reality to cope with mourning	To discuss the possible side-effects, as well as the hypothetical therapeutical application of VR for the treatment of mourning.	-
Quero et al. (2019)	An adaptive virtual reality system for the treatment of adjustment disorder and complicated grief: 1-year follow-up efficacy data.	To examine the long-term efficacy of an adaptive virtual reality system for the treatment of adjustment disorder and complicated grief.	An adaptive virtual reality system

students' perceptions of palliative care; this specifically involved a 27-minute VR lecture on nausea and vomiting management in palliative care and oncology settings and a VR experience of radiotherapy from a patient's viewpoint.

Multidisciplinary collaborations have also benefited from VR technology. Lee et al. (2020) explore the use of a VR platform to promote interprofessional collaboration among healthcare students through team-building activities, team meetings with the patient and family, and team debriefing about the experience. Sanborn et al. (2019) explore the use of simulated palliative and end-of-life care conferences through an online VR environment among healthcare students, while Lee et al. (2020) develop an interprofessional educational experience in a virtual world environment which is found acceptable to graduate participants and results in improved attitudes toward interprofessional education and teamwork after just one virtual session. For an overview of various studies on the use of VR for training and education, please refer to Table 5.10.

Table 5.10 Training and education

First Author	Research Title	Aim	VR Content
Andrade et al. (2010)	Avatar-mediated training in the delivery of bad news in a virtual world.	To study the feasibility of creating SP avatars in a virtual world for the task of training medical trainees to deliver bad news.	Avatar-mediated training
Lee et al. (2020)	The feasibility and acceptability of using virtual world technology for interprofessional education in palliative care: a mixed methods study.	To evaluate the feasibility and acceptability of using a virtual world educational environment for interprofessional health professions students learning about palliative care.	Small-group immersive educational experience focused on palliative care in the virtual world of Second Life®
Hall et al. (2024)	The use of simulated participant and virtual reality simulation to enhance nursing students' communication skills in "end of life care"—a single-arm repeated measures study.	To explore the efficacy of simulation-based learning utilizing VR and simulated participants in a sample of undergraduate nursing students enrolled in a Bachelor of Nursing.	360-degree-video with all the variations and potential outcomes resulting from nursing a person given a life-limiting diagnosis and following that care to death

(*Continued*)

Table 5.10 (Continued)

First Author	Research Title	Aim	VR Content
Sanborn et al. (2019)	Practising interprofessional communication competencies with health profession learners in a palliative care virtual simulation: A curricular short report.	To investigate a 6-week learning activity of using an online virtual reality environment through Second Life® to advance interprofessional education with a convenience sample of undergraduate and graduate health professions learners through a simulated palliative and end-of-life care conference.	Second Life®
Taubert et al. (2019)	Virtual reality videos used in undergraduate palliative and oncology medical teaching: results of a pilot study.	To evaluate whether VR is an effective and acceptable teaching environment.	Pre-recorded 27-minute presentation on nausea and vomiting in palliative care settings
Zhang et al. (2024)	The impact of virtual clinical simulation on nursing students' palliative care knowledge, ability, and attitudes: A mixed methods study.	To develop a virtual clinical simulation education system and assess its impact on enhancing nursing students' knowledge, ability, and attitudes toward palliative care.	1-hour learning session using the virtual clinical simulation education system

Support to Palliative Care Providers

Palliative care providers often experience emotional exhaustion and burnout (Gómez-Urquiza et al., 2020; Parola et al., 2017), resulting in increased rates of staff sickness and absence, compromised patient safety, and poorer quality of patient care (Hall et al., 2016; Parola et al., 2017). VR technology has been preliminarily studied to provide relevant emotional support. For example, Rice et al. (2014) investigate the use of 3D outdoor virtual meetings for peer storytelling sessions to support oncology nurses dealing with grief. In a different approach, Mercante et al. (2024) use a 10-minute session with an immersive meditation experience to support paediatric palliative providers, with the results suggesting this as a feasible and effective approach for mood improvement in palliative care providers. In addition, Dixon et al. (2024) study the use of VR as a therapeutic tool to improve staff well-being in palliative care settings, emphasizing its potential to alleviate stress and enhance job satisfaction. Please refer to Table 5.11 for various studies on using VR to support palliative care providers.

Table 5.11 Support to palliative care providers

First Author	Research Title	Aim	VR Content
Dixon et al. (2024)	VR as a therapeutic tool for palliative and end of life care staff wellbeing.	To explore the use of VR as a resource to support staff during their limited break time and determine its feasibility and impact on areas of wellbeing.	Self-selection among the three VR experiences
Mercante et al. (2024)	Virtual reality intervention as support to pediatric palliative care providers: A pilot study.	To verify immersive virtual reality interventions' feasibility, safety, and efficacy in relieving the psychological distress of PPC staff working in the paediatric hospice.	Ten-minute session of an English demo version of the TRIPP software, created to induce relaxation
Rice et al. (2014)	Using second life to facilitate peer storytelling for grieving oncology nurses.	To investigate the use of a web-based, three-dimensional virtual world technology (Second Life®) that provides a venue to facilitate peer storytelling to support nurses dealing with grief.	Second Life®

Conclusions

This chapter highlights the immense potential of VR for transforming the care and support available for patients, family, and palliative care providers. As every effort is made to help patients live fully until their last moment, a growing body of empirical evidence increasingly supports the efficacy of VR interventions. Moving forward, it is suggested that researchers and clinicians continually explore the full breadth of VR interventions in meeting the specific needs of patients, families, and palliative care providers that traditional interventions may not address.

References

Altman, K., Saredakis, D., Keage, H., Hutchinson, A., Corlis, M., Smith, R. T., Crawford, G. B., & Loetscher, T. (2024). Personalised virtual reality in palliative care: Clinically meaningful symptom improvement for some. *BMJ Supportive & Palliative Care*. https://doi.org/10.1136/spcare-2024-004815

Ando, M., Morita, T., & O'Connor, S. J. (2007). Primary concerns of advanced cancer patients identified through the structured life review process: A qualitative study using a text mining technique. *Palliative and Supportive Care*, 5(3), 265–271. https://doi.org/10.1017/S1478951507000430

Ando, M., Sumitani, M., Sakamura, M., Noguchi, T., Oki, R., Abe, H., Inoue, R., Tsuchida, R., & Uchida, K. (2020). Tele virtual reality-based peer support programme for cancer patients: A preliminary feasibility and acceptability study. *British Journal of Cancer Research*, 3(4), 443–448.

Andrade, A. D., Bagri, A., Zaw, K., Roos, B. A., & Ruiz, J. G. (2010). Avatar-mediated training in the delivery of bad news in a virtual world. *Journal of Palliative Medicine, 13*(12), 1415–1419.

Anekar, A. A., Hendrix, J. M., & Cascella, M. (2023). WHO analgesic ladder. In *StatPearls [Internet]*. StatPearls Publishing. https://www.ncbi.nlm.nih.gov/books/NBK554435/

Austin, P. D., Siddall, P. J., & Lovell, M. R. (2022). Feasibility and acceptability of virtual reality for cancer pain in people receiving palliative care: A randomised cross-over study. *Supportive Care in Cancer, 30*(5), 3995–4005.

Baños, R. M., Espinoza, M., García-Palacios, A., Cervera, J. M., Esquerdo, G., Barrajón, E., & Botella, C. (2013). A positive psychological intervention using virtual reality for patients with advanced cancer in a hospital setting: A pilot study to assess feasibility. *Supportive Care in Cancer, 21*, 263–270.

Botella, C., Osma, J., Palacios, A. G., Guillén, V., & Baños, R. (2008). Treatment of complicated grief using virtual reality: A case report. *Death Studies, 32*(7), 674–692. https://doi.org/10.1080/07481180802231319

Brungardt, A., Wibben, A., Shanbhag, P., Boeldt, D., Youngwerth, J., Tompkins, A., Rolbiecki, A. J., Coats, H., LaGasse, A. B., Kutner, J. S., & Lum, H. D. (2024). Patient outcomes of a virtual reality-based music therapy pilot in palliative care. *Palliative Medicine Reports, 5*(1), 278–285. https://doi.org/10.1089/pmr.2024.0022

Brungardt, A., Wibben, A., Tompkins, A. F., Shanbhag, P., Coats, H., LaGasse, A. B., Boeldt, D., Youngwerth, J., Kutner, J. S., & Lum, H. D. (2021). Virtual reality-based music therapy in palliative care: A pilot implementation trial. *Journal of Palliative Medicine, 24*(5), 736–742.

Burridge, N., Sillence, A., Teape, L., Clark, B., Bruce, E., Armoogum, J., Leloch, D., Spathis, A., & Etkind, S. (2023). Virtual reality reduces anxiety and pain in acute hospital palliative care: Service evaluation. *BMJ Supportive & Palliative Care*. https://doi.org/10.1136/spcare-2023-004572

Carmont, H., & McIlfatrick, S. (2022). Using virtual reality in palliative care: A systematic integrative review. *International Journal of Palliative Nursing, 28*(3), 132–144.

Chang, Y.-K., Wu, Y.-K., & Liu, T.-H. (2024). The effectiveness of a virtual reality teaching module on advance care planning and advance decision for medical professionals. *BMC Medical Education, 24*(1), 112. https://doi.org/10.1186/s12909-023-04990-y

Corvin, J., Hoskinson, Z., Mozolic-Staunton, B., Hattingh, L., & Plumbridge-Jones, R. (2024). The effects of virtual reality interventions on occupational participation and distress from symptoms in palliative care patients: A pilot study. *Palliative & Supportive Care*, 1–8. https://doi.org/10.1017/S1478951524000245

Dang, M., Noreika, D., Ryu, S., Sima, A., Ashton, H., Ondris, B., Coley, F., Nestler, J., & Fabbro, E. D. (2021). Feasibility of delivering an avatar-facilitated life review intervention for patients with cancer. *Journal of Palliative Medicine, 24*(4), 520–526.

Deeken, A. (2004). Life meets death; east meets west. In *Hong Kong society of palliative medicine newsletter* (Vol. 3, pp. 4–8). End of life/Palliative Education Resource Centre.

Deming, J. R., Dunbar, K. J., Lueck, J. F., & Oh, Y. (2024). Virtual reality videos for symptom management in hospice and palliative care. *Mayo Clinic Proceedings: Digital Health*. https://doi.org/10.1016/j.mcpdig.2024.08.002

Dixon, E., Tilki, B., Pereira, L., Pearlman, D., Marsh, I., Rodrigues, M., Collis, E., Bennetts, J., & Tavabie, S. (2024). 44 VR as a therapeutic tool for palliative and end of life care staff wellbeing. *BMJ Supportive & Palliative Care, 14*(Suppl. 2), A24–A25. https://doi.org/10.1136/spcare-2024-PCC.62

Ferguson, C., Shade, M. Y., Blaskewicz Boron, J., Lyden, E., & Manley, N. A. (2020). Virtual reality for therapeutic recreation in dementia hospice care: A feasibility study. *American Journal of Hospice and Palliative Medicine®, 37*(10), 809–815.

Filho, B. A. B. D. S., & Tritany, É. F. (2022). Immersive virtual reality in palliative care: Prospects for total rehabilitation. *Cadernos de Terapia Ocupacional Da UFS-Car, 30*, 1–13. https://doi.org/10.1590/2526-8910.ctoARF22923024

Fitzsimons, D., Mullan, D., Wilson, J. S., Conway, B., Corcoran, B., Dempster, M., Gamble, J., Stewart, C., Rafferty, S., McMahon, M., MacMahon, J., Mulholland, P., Stockdale, P., Chew, E., Hanna, L., Brown, J., Ferguson, G., & Fogarty, D. (2007). The challenge of patients' unmet palliative care needs in the final stages of chronic illness. *Palliative Medicine, 21*(4), 313–322. https://doi.org/10.1177/0269216307077711

Gaggioli, A., Bassi, M., & Delle Fave, A. (2003). Quality of experience in virtual environments. In G. Riva, W. IJsselsteijn, & F. Davide (Eds.), *Being there: Concepts, effects and measurement of user presence in synthetic environments* (pp. 121–135). IOS Press.

Gerlach, C., Greinacher, A., Alt-Epping, B., & Wrzus, C. (2023). My virtual home: Needs of patients in palliative cancer care and content effects of individualized virtual reality—a mixed methods study protocol. *BMC Palliative Care, 22*(1), 1–167. https://doi.org/10.1186/s12904-023-01297-z

Gómez-Urquiza, J. L., Albendín-García, L., Velando-Soriano, A., Ortega-Campos, E., Ramírez-Baena, L., Membrive-Jiménez, M. J., & Suleiman-Martos, N. (2020). Burnout in palliative care nurses, prevalence and risk factors: A systematic review with meta-analysis. *International Journal of Environmental Research and Public Health, 17*(20), 7672. https://doi.org/10.3390/ijerph17207672

Groninger, H., Stewart, D., Fisher, J. M., Tefera, E., Cowgill, J., & Mete, M. (2021). Virtual reality for pain management in advanced heart failure: A randomized controlled study. *Palliative Medicine, 35*(10), 2008–2016.

Guenther, M., Görlich, D., Bernhardt, F., Pogatzki-Zahn, E., Dasch, B., Krueger, J., & Lenz, P. (2022). Virtual reality reduces pain in palliative care–a feasibility trial. *BMC Palliative Care, 21*(1), 169.

Hall, K., Bhowmik, J., Simonda, I., & Edward, K. (2024). The use of simulated participant and virtual reality simulation to enhance nursing students' communication skills in "end of life care"—a single-arm repeated measures study. *Clinical Simulation in Nursing, 91*, 101543. https://doi.org/10.1016/j.ecns.2024.101543

Hall, L. H., Johnson, J., Watt, I., Tsipa, A., & O'Connor, D. B. (2016). Healthcare staff wellbeing, burnout, and patient safety: A systematic review. *PloS One, 11*(7), e0159015. https://doi.org/10.1371/journal.pone.0159015

Hartshorn, G., Browning, M., Chalil Madathil, K., Mau, F., Ranganathan, S., Todd, A., Bertrand, J., Maynard, A., McAnirlin, O., Sindelar, K., Hernandez, R., & Henry Gomez, T. (2022). Efficacy of virtual reality assisted guided imagery (VRAGI) in a home setting for pain management in patients with advanced cancer: Protocol for a randomised controlled trial. *BMJ Open, 12*(12), e064363. https://doi.org/10.1136/bmjopen-2022-064363

Hoffman, A. J., Brintnall, R. A., Brown, J. K., Von Eye, A., Jones, L. W., Alderink, G., Ritz-Holland, D., Enter, M., Patzelt, L. H., & VanOtteren, G. M. (2014). Virtual reality bringing a new reality to postthoracotomy lung cancer patients via a home-based exercise intervention targeting fatigue while undergoing adjuvant treatment. *Cancer Nursing, 37*(1), 23–33.

Houska, A., & Loučka, M. (2019). Patients' autonomy at the end of life: A critical review. *Journal of Pain and Symptom Management, 57*(4), 835–845. https://doi.org/10.1016/j.jpainsymman.2018.12.339

Hsieh, W. T. (2020). Virtual reality video promotes effectiveness in advance care planning. *BMC Palliative Care, 19*, 1–10. https://doi.org/10.1186/s12904-020-00634-w

Huang, Y., Deng, C., Peng, M., & Hao, Y. (2024). Experiences and perceptions of palliative care patients receiving virtual reality therapy: A meta-synthesis of qualitative studies. *BMC Palliative Care, 23*(1), 182. https://doi.org/10.1186/s12904-024-01520-5

Irving, H. (2023). Virtual reality gives hospice patients the experiences they long for. *Canadian Healthcare Technology, 28*(8), 4.

Jacobsen, R., Møldrup, C., Christrup, L., & Sjøgren, P. (2009). Patient-related barriers to cancer pain management: A systematic exploratory review. *Scandinavian Journal of Caring Sciences, 23*(1), 190–208. https://doi.org/10.1111/j.1471-6712.2008.00601.x

Johnson, T., Bauler, L., Vos, D., Hifko, A., Garg, P., Ahmed, M., & Raphelson, M. (2020). Virtual reality use for symptom management in palliative care: A pilot study to assess user perceptions. *Journal of Palliative Medicine, 23*(9), 1233–1238. https://doi.org/10.1089/jpm.2019.0411

Kelleher, S. A., Fisher, H. M., Winger, J. G., Miller, S. N., Amaden, G. H., Somers, T. J., Colloca, L., Uronis, H. E., & Keefe, F. J. (2022). Virtual reality for improving pain and pain-related symptoms in patients with advanced stage colorectal cancer: A pilot trial to test feasibility and acceptability. *Palliative & Supportive Care, 20*(4), 471–481.

Kiernat, J. (1979). The use of life review activity with confused nursing home residents. *American Journal of Occupational Therapy, 33*(5), 306–310.

Kim, H., & Flieger, S. P. (2023). Barriers to effective communication about advance care planning and palliative care: A qualitative study. *Journal of Hospice and Palliative Care, 26*(2), 42–50. https://doi.org/10.14475/jhpc.2023.26.2.42

Knowles, L. M., Stelzer, E.-M., Jovel, K. S., & O'Connor, M.-F. (2017). A pilot study of virtual support for grief: Feasibility, acceptability, and preliminary outcomes. *Computers in Human Behavior, 73*, 650–658. https://doi.org/10.1016/j.chb.2017.04.005

Laffer, A., Corle, M., Canell, A., Moo, L., Gately, M., & Dillon, K. (2023). Implementation of virtual reality to improve quality of life for veterans in hospice and palliative care. *Innovation in Aging, 7*(Suppl. 1), 1064–1065. https://doi.org/10.1093/geroni/igad104.3420

Lee, A. L., DeBest, M., Koeniger-Donohue, R., Strowman, S. R., & Mitchell, S. E. (2020). The feasibility and acceptability of using virtual world technology for interprofessional education in palliative care: A mixed methods study. *Journal of Interprofessional Care, 34*(4), 461–471. https://doi.org/10.1080/13561820.2019.1643832

Liao, D., Xia, Y., Xu, M., & Ding, M. (2023). A grief farewell scene design for children based on virtual reality. In *International conference on artificial intelligence and industrial design (AIID 2022)* (Vol. 12612, p. 126120G). https://doi.org/10.1117/12.2673048

Lloyd, A., & Haraldsdottir, E. (2021). Virtual reality in hospice: Improved patient well-being. *BMJ Supportive & Palliative Care, 11*(3), 344–350.

Lombard, M., & Ditton, T. (1997). At the heart of it all: The concept of presence. *Journal of Computer-Mediated Communication, 3*(2), 20.

Mackey, B. A., Bremner, P. A., & Giuliani, M. (2020, March). Immersive control of a robot surrogate for users in palliative care. In *Companion of the 2020 ACM/IEEE international conference on human-robot interaction* (pp. 585–587). https://doi.org/10.1145/3371382.3377445

Maddox, T., Oldstone, L., Sparks, C. Y., Sackman, J., Oyao, A., Garcia, L., Maddox, R. U., Ffrench, K., Garcia, H., Adair, T., Irvin, A., Maislin, D., Keenan, B., Bonakdar, R., & Darnall, B. D. (2023). In-home virtual reality program for chronic lower back pain: A randomized Sham-controlled effectiveness trial in a clinically severe and diverse sample. *Mayo Clinic Proceedings: Digital Health, 1*(4), 563–573. https://doi.org/10.1016/j.mcpdig.2023.09.003

Martin, J. L., Saredakis, D., Hutchinson, A. D., Crawford, G. B., & Loetscher, T. (2022). Virtual reality in palliative care: A systematic review. *Healthcare (Basel), 10*(7), 1222.

Mercante, A., Zanin, A., Vecchi, L., De Tommasi, V., & Benini, F. (2024). Virtual reality intervention as support to paediatric palliative care providers: A pilot study. *Acta Paediatrica, 113*(4), 833–834. https://doi.org/10.1111/apa.17099

Mo, J., Vickerstaff, V., Minton, O., Tavabie, S., Taubert, M., Stone, P., & White, N. (2022). How effective is virtual reality technology in palliative care? A systematic review and meta-analysis. *Palliative Medicine, 36*(7), 1047–1058.

Mohammad, E. B., & Ahmad, M. (2019). Virtual reality as a distraction technique for pain and anxiety among patients with breast cancer: A randomized control trial. *Palliative & Supportive Care, 17*(1), 29–34.

Moloney, M., Doody, O., O'Reilly, M., Lucey, M., Callinan, J., Exton, C., Colreavy, S., O'Mahony, F., Meskell, P., & Coffey, A. (2023). Virtual reality use and patient outcomes in palliative care: A scoping review. *Digital Health, 9*, 20552076231207576. https://doi.org/10.1177/20552076231207574

Moon, N. O., Henstridge-Blows, J. R., Sprecher, E. A., Thomas, E., Byfield, A., & McGrane, J. (2023). 'Godrevy project': Virtual reality for symptom control and well-being in oncology and palliative care—a non-randomised pre-post interventional trial. *BMJ Oncology, 2*(1), e000160. https://doi.org/10.1136/bmjonc-2023-000160

Moscato, S., Sichi, V., Giannelli, A., Palumbo, P., Ostan, R., & Chiari, L. (2021). Virtual reality in home palliative care: Brief report on the effect on cancer-related symptomatology. *Frontiers in Psychology, 12*, 709154.

Moutogiannis, P. P., Thrift, J., Pope, J. K., Browning, M. H. E. M., McAnirlin, O., & Fasolino, T. (2023). A rapid review of the role of virtual reality in care delivery of palliative care and hospice. *Journal of Hospice and Palliative Nursing, 25*(6), 300–308. https://doi.org/10.1097/NJH.0000000000000983

Mukai, T., Tsukiyama, Y., Yamada, S., Nishikawa, A., Hayami, S., Noguchi, R., Yoshida, J., Kashiwada, M., Ohta, S., Shimokawa, T., & Yamaue, H. (2023). Virtual reality images of the home are useful for patients with hospital-based palliative care: Prospective observational study with analysis by text mining. *Palliative Medicine Reports, 4*(1), 214–219. https://doi.org/10.1089/pmr.2023.0017

Nagelschmidt, K., Leppin, N., Seifart, C., Rief, W., & von Blanckenburg, P. (2021). Systematic mixed-method review of barriers to end-of-life communication in the family context. *BMJ Supportive & Palliative Care, 11*(3), 253–263. https://doi.org/10.1136/bmjspcare-2020-002219

Ng, R., Woo, K. L. O., Eckhoff, D., Zhu, M., Lee, A., & Cassinelli, A. (2024). Participatory design of a virtual reality life review therapy system for palliative care. *Frontiers in Virtual Reality, 5*. https://doi.org/10.3389/frvir.2024.1304615

Niki, K., Egashira, S., & Okamoto, Y. (2024). A real-time virtual outing using virtual reality for a hospitalized terminal cancer patient who has difficulty going out: A case report. *Frontiers in Virtual Reality, 5.* https://doi.org/10.3389/frvir.2024.1269707

Niki, K., Okamoto, Y., Maeda, I., Mori, I., Ishii, R., Matsuda, Y., Takagi, T., & Uejima, E. (2019). A novel palliative care approach using virtual reality for improving various symptoms of terminal cancer patients: A preliminary prospective, multicenter study. *Journal of Palliative Medicine, 22*(6), 72–707.

Nwosu, A. C., Mills, M., Roughneen, S., Stanley, S., Chapman, L., & Mason, S. R. (2024). Virtual reality in specialist palliative care: A feasibility study to enable clinical practice adoption. *BMJ Supportive & Palliative Care, 14*(1), 47–51.

O'Philbin, L., Woods, B., Farrell, E. M., Spector, A. E., & Orrell, M. (2018). Reminiscence therapy for dementia: An abridged Cochrane systematic review of the evidence from randomized controlled trials. *Expert Review of Neurotherapeutics, 18*(9), 715–727.

Ouchi, K. (2023). Virtual reality for palliative care communication training: A novel dissemination strategy. *Innovation in Aging, 7*(Suppl. 1), 325. https://doi.org/10.1093/geroni/igad104.1083

Park, K., Lee, S., Yang, J., Song, T., & Hong, G.-R. S. (2019). A systematic review and meta-analysis on the effect of reminiscence therapy for people with dementia. *International Psychogeriatrics, 31*(11), 1581–1597.

Parola, V., Coelho, A., Cardoso, D., Sandgren, A., & Apóstolo, J. (2017). Prevalence of burnout in health professionals working in palliative care: A systematic review. *JBI Database of Systematic Reviews and Implementation Reports, 15*(7), 1905–1933. https://doi.org/10.11124/jbisrir-2016-003309

Perna, L., Lund, S., White, N., & Minton, O. (2021). The potential of personalized virtual reality in palliative care: A feasibility trial. *American Journal of Hospice and Palliative Medicine®, 38*(12), 1488–1494.

Pizzoli, S. F. M., Monzani, D., Vergani, L., Sanchini, V., & Mazzocco, K. (2023). From virtual to real healing: A critical overview of the therapeutic use of virtual reality to cope with mourning. *Current Psychology (New Brunswick, N.J.), 42*(11), 8697–8704. https://doi.org/10.1007/s12144-021-02158-9

Quero, S., Molés, M., Campos, D., Andreu-Mateu, S., Baños, R. M., & Botella, C. (2019). An adaptive virtual reality system for the treatment of adjustment disorder and complicated grief: 1-year follow-up efficacy data. *Clinical Psychology and Psychotherapy, 26*(2), 204–217. https://doi.org/10.1002/cpp.2342

Rice, K. L., Bennett, M. J., & Billingsley, L. (2014). Using second life to facilitate peer storytelling for grieving oncology nurses. *Ochsner Journal, 14*(4), 551–562.

Ritchie, C. S., & Kotwal, A. A. (2023). Loneliness and social isolation in palliative care: A call to action. *Journal of Palliative Medicine, 26*(8), 1032–1034. https://doi.org/10.1089/jpm.2023.0425

Ryu, S., & Price, S. K. (2022). Embodied storytelling and meaning-making at the end of life: VoicingHan avatar life-review for palliative care in cancer patients. *Arts & Health, 14*(3), 326–340.

Sanborn, H., Cole, J., Kennedy, T., & Saewert, K. J. (2019). Practicing interprofessional communication competencies with health profession learners in a palliative care virtual simulation: A curricular short report. *Journal of Interprofessional Education & Practice, 15*, 48–54.

Saunders, C. M. (1967). *The management of terminal malignant disease* (1st ed.). Hospital Medicine Publications.

Tan, A., Ross, S. P., & Duerksen, K. (2013). Death is not always a failure: Outcomes from implementing an online virtual patient clinical case in palliative care for family medicine clerkship. *Medical Education Online*, *18*(1), 22711.

Taubert, M., Webber, L., Hamilton, T., Carr, M., & Harvey, M. (2019). Virtual reality videos used in undergraduate palliative and oncology medical teaching: Results of a pilot study. *BMJ Supportive & Palliative Care*, *9*(3), 281–285.

Vasudevan, A. V., Cao, Y., Gough, P., & Ahmadpour, N. (2023). Enrichment through virtual reality for palliative care: A scoping review. In *Proceedings of the 35th Australian computer-human interaction conference* (pp. 280–293). https://doi.org/10.1145/3638380.3638389

Wang, C. W., Chow, A. Y., & Chan, C. L. (2017). The effects of life review interventions on spiritual well-being, psychological distress, and quality of life in patients with terminal or advanced cancer: A systematic review and meta-analysis of randomized controlled trials. *Palliative Medicine*, *31*(10), 883–894. https://doi.org/10.1177/0269216317705101

Warth, M., Kessler, J., Koehler, F., Aguilar-Raab, C., Bardenheuer, H., & Ditzen, B. (2019). Brief psychosocial interventions improve quality of life of patients receiving palliative care: A systematic review and meta-analysis. *Palliative Medicine*, *33*(3), 332–345.

Weingarten, K., Macapagal, F., & Parker, D. (2020). Virtual reality: Endless potential in pediatric palliative care: A case report. *Journal of Palliative Medicine*, *23*(1), 147–149.

Wong, C. L., Li, C. K., Chan, C. W. H., Choi, K. C., Chen, J., Yeung, M. T., & Chan, O. N. (2021). Virtual reality intervention targeting pain and anxiety among pediatric cancer patients undergoing peripheral intravenous cannulation: A randomized controlled trial. *Cancer Nursing*, *44*(6), 435–442. https://doi.org/10.1097/NCC.0000000000000844

Wong, C. L., Li, C. K., Choi, K. C., Wei So, W. K., Yan Kwok, J. Y., Cheung, Y. T., & Chan, C. W. H. (2022). Effects of immersive virtual reality for managing anxiety, nausea and vomiting among paediatric cancer patients receiving their first chemotherapy: An exploratory randomised controlled trial. *European Journal of Oncology Nursing: The Official Journal of European Oncology Nursing Society*, *61*, 102233. https://doi.org/10.1016/j.ejon.2022.102233

Woo, O. K. L., & Lee, A. M. (2023). Case report: Therapeutic potential of flourishing-life-of-wish virtual reality therapy on relaxation (FLOW-VRT-relaxation)—a novel personalized relaxation in palliative care. *Frontiers in Digital Health*, *5*. https://doi.org/10.3389/fdgth.2023.1228781

Woo, O. K. L., Lee, A. M., Ng, R., Eckhoff, D., Lo, R., & Cassinelli, A. (2024). Flourishing-life-of-wish virtual reality relaxation therapy (FLOW-VRT-relaxation) outperforms traditional relaxation therapy in palliative care: Results from a randomized controlled trial. *Frontiers in Virtual Reality*, *4*, 1304155.

Zhang, L., Huang, Y., Wu, X., Liu, C., Zhang, X., Yang, X., Lai, H., Fu, J., & Yang, M. (2024). The impact of virtual clinical simulation on nursing students' palliative care knowledge, ability, and attitudes: A mixed methods study. *Nurse Education Today*, *132*, 106037. https://doi.org/10.1016/j.nedt.2023.106037

6 Theoretical Foundations for Using Virtual Reality in Palliative Care

Introduction

While emerging scientific evidence supports the efficacy of VR in symptom management, the literature appears to lack robust theoretical frameworks for its application in palliative care. This chapter seeks to explore and elaborate on relevant psychological theories that may enhance our understanding of the potential benefits and applications of VR for patients with terminal illnesses. These theories include flow, restoration, self-determination, and stress-coping theories. It is hoped that these theoretical insights will facilitate future research and clinical practice, ensuring that VR interventions are grounded in both empirical evidence and theoretical principles.

Flow Theory

Flow refers to a psychological state in which a person has a sense of control but without reflective self-consciousness (Engeser et al., 2021). It is characterized by full absorption in an activity that one hardly thinks of oneself or current states during flow experience (Chen, 2007). It is described as an "optimal experience" when the person feels happy, motivated, and cognitively efficient (Moneta & Csikszentmihalyi, 1996). Flow is associated with positive affect (Abuhamdeh, 2021), with greater flow corresponding to a greater positive affect in the context of VR (Cheng et al., 2014). Neurophysiological findings link the flow experience with dopamine receptor availability (de Manzano et al., 2013; Gyurkovics et al., 2016), indicating flow as an enjoyable state.

Flow has been shown to bring physical and psychological benefits. Research has found that the physical health of elderly Japanese individuals is significantly better among those who report experiencing flow or a relaxed state when performing daily activities compared to those in an apathetic state (Hirao et al., 2012). The positive emotion and focused attention associated with flow have been proposed to alter pain experiences (Villemure &

DOI: 10.4324/9781003518327-9

Bushnell, 2002). Among older adults, flow has also been linked to subjective well-being, life satisfaction, physical health, and mental health (Heo et al., 2010a, 2010b, 2013), which highlights flow as a potential underlying mechanism in the management of both physical and emotional symptoms.

VR has been associated with flow and appraised as a flow-inducing technology, as it can enrich human experiences through sensory stimulations such as sight, sound, and touch. Gaggioli et al. (2003) point out four crucial characteristics of VR that suggest its potential effectiveness in fostering flow. First, situations and tasks can be designed in the virtual environment such that the individual can begin with the simplest situations and move towards more complicated tasks. Second, the virtual tasks require specific skills, such as cognitive and practical ones, that can be refined and gradually increased during the sessions. Third, VR systems can offer multimodal feedback to individuals' actions and behaviour. Fourth, individuals can experience control of the situation while interacting in the virtual world and using their abilities.

The physical limitations that many patients in palliative care face often hinder their ability to engage in meaningful activities, which can restrict their potential to experience flow. Although behavioural activation interventions aim to enhance mood through active participation (Veale, 2008), these approaches are frequently challenged by the patients' physical constraints and bedbound conditions. In contrast, VR technology presents a promising alternative that can facilitate flow experiences, enabling patients to engage in activities that may be physically demanding or impossible in the real world. This unique aspect of VR not only mitigates the impact of physical limitations but also allows patients to harness their cognitive and learning skills in a virtual and controlled setting. It may eventually enhance their physical and emotional well-being and promote positive engagement through innovative therapeutic avenues.

Attention Restoration Theory

Restoration or restorativeness refers to the renewal of physical and psychological resources depleted in continual efforts to meet the demands of daily life (Hartig & Staats, 2003; Parsons & Hartig, 2000). It serves to improve sustained attention (Hartig et al., 1991), reduce stress (Ulrich, 1983), and foster positive emotions (Hartig et al., 1999). Kaplan (1995, 2001) distinguished between two types of attention. *Directed attention* refers to a type of attention that requires effort, concentration, and sustained focus. It is described as a "top-down" process, more linked to higher-order cognitive functions such as working memory and problem-solving. Such continual effort and concentration may lead to "directed attention fatigue." If directed attention fatigue is not well resolved, it results in negative consequences, such as poorer decision-making, lower levels of self-control (Hare et al., 2009; Vohs et al., 2008), and negative psychological state, such as feeling irritable and uncomfortable (De Young, 2007). In contrast, *involuntary attention* is driven by curiosity, fascination, and exploration. It is spontaneous and effortless, being able to alleviate the directed attention fatigue and restore one's well-being.

In the context of cancer, abundant research has investigated the application of restoration to improve patient's well-being. The "natural restorative environmental interventions" have been shown to bring beneficial effects (Berto et al., 2010; Korpela et al., 2008; Norling et al., 2008; Staats et al., 2010, Jung et al., 2017). It refers to various formats of interventions that capitalize on the restorative function of the natural environment and have been tested efficacious in improving attention in different populations (Kaplan & Berman, 2010). Examples include nature tasks, such as gardening and walking, among women with early breast cancer (Cimprich & Ronis, 2003) and viewing nature pictures on a computer display among college students (Berman et al., 2008).

In light of the restorative functions, VR appears to have unlimited potential to facilitate restorative and stress-reducing effects in constrained patients, such as those who are confined in the hospital walls in a palliative care setting. The study by Scates et al. (2020) finds that VR nature view significantly increases relaxation, feelings of peace, and positive distractions among cancer patients. Wilkie and Stavridou (2013) report that VR produces a restorative effect, especially for those who cannot access natural environments. A systematic review (Riches et al., 2021) supports that the combination of natural audio-visual features can activate the parasympathetic system, thereby facilitating relaxation, mood regulation, and stress recovery. This is particularly relevant for patients with terminal illnesses, who are often exhausted by the directed attention required to cope with their terminal illnesses and whose hospital environments may have limited capacity for activities that engage in activities that facilitate involuntary attention.

Self-Determination Theory

Self-determination theory emphasizes the central role of the individual's inner resources for personality development and behavioural self-regulation, highlighting human motivation and personality functioning (Deci & Ryan, 1985, 2000; Ryan & Deci, 2000, 2002, 2022). It proposes that an individual is growth-oriented and driven to actualize his or her potentialities. An individual's behaviour is often triggered by intrinsic motivation, which is a form of motivation intrinsic in nature, such as an enjoyable and captivating experience, in contrast to extrinsic motivation that is driven by an external goal, such as garnering praise and approval (Ryan & Deci, 2017). Such principles that facilitate self-initiated behaviour have been applied in different aspects, such as promoting changes in health behaviour (Gillison et al., 2019), facilitating learning in schools (Guay, 2022), enhancing persistence in sports and exercises (Standage & Ryan, 2020), and maintaining effects of psychotherapy (Ryan et al., 2011).

Self-determination theory also proposes the active development and integration that happens along with the constant fulfillment of basic psychological needs, such as autonomy, competence, and relatedness (Ryan & Deci, 2022). *Autonomy* refers to the ability to make independent choices with support from the environment. *Competence* refers to the ability to influence the environment, whereas *relatedness* refers to the perceived connection or support an individual receives from other people in the environment (Standage & Ryan, 2020). The meta-analysis by Cerasoli and colleagues (2016) finds that autonomy, competence, and relatedness are predictors of qualitative performance, such as creativity, user experience, and technical sophistication. In contrast, individuals with unfulfilled basic psychological needs tend to suffer from poorer psychological health at work (Trépanier et al., 2013).

VR's capability for personalization may help fulfill the self-determination needs of patients by allowing them to choose their preferred virtual content. The study of Gerlach and colleagues (2024) finds that personalized content created for patients under palliative care based on their individual choices significantly improves their levels of tiredness and calmness. A randomized controlled trial conducted by Woo et al. (2024) reports the outperforming performance of VR psychological interventions, which allows patients to choose their preferred virtual content for relaxation over traditional relaxation therapy with a greater reduction in physical and psychological symptoms in the VR group. The personalization feature of VR appears to support the basic psychological needs of autonomy through personal choice of VR content, competence through facilitating their use of the novel device, and relatedness through encouraging user's expression of their emotions or intentions (Oulasvirta & Blom, 2008).

Stress Coping Theory

Coping refers to the dynamic cognitive and behavioural strategies used to manage specific external and internal demands that are perceived as taxing or exceeding an individual's resources (Lazarus & Folkman, 1984). Their theory of cognitive appraisal, stress, and coping distinguishes between two ways of coping with stress. *Problem-focused coping* refers to a coping style that focuses on controlling the current stressful situation by modifying, avoiding, or reducing the influences of a stressor. *Emotion-focused coping* aims to manage one's emotions in response to a stressor. Although a person can adopt either coping style in the face of a stressful event, he or she tends to adopt emotion-focused coping when the stressful condition cannot be easily resolved, such as suffering from a terminal illness, whereas curative treatment is no longer an option.

VR technology may facilitate emotion-focused coping in patients who encounter incurable illnesses through the rehabilitation journey. Johnson et al. (2020) deliver one 30-minute VR session to adult hospice patients, who find the VR experience mostly enjoyable and pleasant, with some requesting more VR sessions. Similar results are obtained in the study of Ferguson et al. (2020), which shows that most hospice patients with dementia enjoy using VR for therapeutic recreation. Such evidence may be explained by the inherent enjoyment offered by VR, which is facilitated by the sense of presence brought by the immersive experience. With more pleasure derived from using VR, users are more willing to participate in VR activity (Buche et al., 2022; Rose et al., 2018).

Conclusions

This chapter introduces the psychological theories that potentially underpin the therapeutic benefits of using VR technology in palliative care. The empirical evidence related to its application in the context of palliative care has been reviewed, supporting the idea that this technology can be theoretically grounded and complement traditional interventions in end-of-life care. However, further research is essential to develop and strengthen the theoretical foundations that can guide the design and implementation of VR-based interventions. It is hoped that this chapter serves as a valuable starting point from a psychological perspective while also encouraging the investigation of additional frameworks that warrant further research.

References

Abuhamdeh, S. (2021). On the relationship between flow and enjoyment. In *Advances in flow research* (pp. 155–169). Springer International Publishing. https://doi.org/10.1007/978-3-030-53468-4_6

Berman, M. G., Jonides, J., & Kaplan, S. (2008). The cognitive benefits of interacting with nature. *Psychological Science, 19*(12), 1207–1212. https://doi.org/10.1111/j.1467-9280.2008.02225.x

Berto, R., Baroni, M. R., Zainaghi, A., & Bettella, S. (2010). An exploratory study of the effect of high and low fascination environments on attentional fatigue. *Journal of Environmental Psychology, 30*(4), 494–500.

Buche, H., Michel, A., & Blanc, N. (2022). Use of virtual reality in oncology: From the state of the art to an integrative model. *Frontiers in Virtual Reality, 3*. https://doi.org/10.3389/frvir.2022.894162

Cerasoli, C. P., Nicklin, J. M., & Nassrelgrgawi, A. S. (2016). Performance, incentives, and needs for autonomy, competence, and relatedness: A meta-analysis. *Motivation and Emotion, 40*(6), 781–813. https://doi.org/10.1007/s11031-016-9578-2

Chen, J. (2007). Flow in games (and everything else). In *Communications of the ACM* (Vol. 50, No. 4, pp. 31–34). Association for Computing Machinery. https://doi.org/10.1145/1232743.1232769

Cheng, L., Chieng, M., & Chieng, W. (2014). Measuring virtual experience in a three-dimensional virtual reality interactive simulator environment: A structural equation modeling approach. *Virtual Reality: The Journal of the Virtual Reality Society, 18*(3), 173–188.

Cimprich, B., & Ronis, D. L. (2003). An environmental intervention to restore attention in women with newly diagnosed breast cancer. *Cancer Nursing, 26*(4), 284–292. https://doi.org/10.1097/00002820-200308000-00005

de Manzano, Ö., Cervenka, S., Jucaite, A., Hellenäs, O., Farde, L., & Ullén, F. (2013). Individual differences in the proneness to have flow experiences are linked to dopamine D2-receptor availability in the dorsal striatum. *NeuroImage, 67*, 1–6. https://doi.org/10.1016/j.neuroimage.2012.10.072

De Young, R. (2007). *Walking for mental vitality: Some psychological benefits of walking in natural settings.* https://www.researchgate.net/publication/251940530_Walking_for_Mental_Vitality_Some_Psychological_Benefits_of_Walking_in_Natural_Settings

Deci, E. L., & Ryan, R. M. (1985). *Intrinsic motivation and self-determination in human behavior.* Plenum.

Deci, E. L., & Ryan, R. M. (2000). The "what" and "why" of goal pursuits: Human needs and the self-determination of behavior. *PsychologicalInquiry, 11*, 227–268.

Engeser, S., Schiepe-Tiska, A., & Peifer, C. (2021). Historical lines and an overview of current research on flow. In *Advances in flow research* (pp. 1–29). Springer International Publishing. https://doi.org/10.1007/978-3-030-53468-4_1

Ferguson, C., Shade, M. Y., Blaskewicz Boron, J., Lyden, E., & Manley, N. A. (2020). Virtual reality for therapeutic recreation in dementia hospice care: A feasibility study. *American Journal of Hospice & Palliative Medicine, 37*(10), 809–815. https://doi.org/10.1177/1049909120901525

Gaggioli, A., Bassi, M., & Delle Fave, A. (2003). Quality of experience in virtual environments. In G. Riva, W. IJsselsteijn, & F. Davide (Eds.), *Being there: Concepts, effects and measurement of user presence in synthetic environments* (pp. 121–135). IOS Press.

Gerlach, C., Haas, L., Greinacher, A., Lantelme, J., Guenther, M., Thiesbonenkamp-Maag, J., alt-Epping, B., & Wrzus, C. (2024). My virtual escape from patient life: A feasibility study on the experiences and benefits of individualized virtual reality for inpatients in palliative cancer care. *Research Square.* https://doi.org/10.21203/rs.3.rs-4565417/v1

Gillison, F. B., Rouse, P., Standage, M., Sebire, S. J., & Ryan, R. M. (2019). A meta-analysis of techniques to promote motivation for health behaviour change from a self-determination theory perspective. *Health Psychology Review, 13*(1), 110–130. https://doi.org/10.1080/17437199.2018.1534071

Guay, F. (2022). Applying self-determination theory to education: Regulations types, psychological needs, and autonomy supporting behaviors. *Canadian Journal of School Psychology, 37*(1), 75–92. https://doi.org/10.1177/08295735211055355

Gyurkovics, M., Kotyuk, E., Katonai, E. R., Horvath, E. Z., Vereczkei, A., & Szekely, A. (2016). Individual differences in flow proneness are linked to a dopamine D2 receptor gene variant. *Consciousness and Cognition, 42*, 1–8. https://doi.org/10.1016/j.concog.2016.02.014

Hare, T. A., Camerer, C. F., & Rangel, A. (2009). Self-control in decision-making involves modulation of the vmpfc valuation system. *Science (American Association for the Advancement of Science)*, *324*(5927), 646–648.

Hartig, T., Mang, M., & Evans, G. W. (1991). Restorative effects of natural environment experiences. *Environment and Behavior, 23,* 3–26.

Hartig, T., Nyberg, L., Nilsson, L. G., & Garling, T. (1999). Testing for mood congruent recall with environmentally induced mood. *Journal of Environmental Psychology, 19,* 353–367.

Hartig, T., & Staats, H. (2003). Guest editors' introduction: Restorative environments. *Journal of Environmental Psychology, 23,* 103–108.

Heo, J., Lee, Y., McCormick, B. P., & Pedersen, P. M. (2010a). Daily experience of serious leisure, flow and subjective wellbeing of older adults. *Leisure Studies, 29*(2), 207–225.

Heo, J., Lee, Y., Pedersen, P. M., & McCormick, B. P. (2010b). Flow experience in the daily lives of older adults: An analysis of the interaction between flow, individual differences, serious leisure, location, and social context. *Canadian Journal on Aging/La Revue Canadienne Du Vieillissement, 29*(3), 411–423.

Heo, J., Stebbins, R. A., Kim, J., & Lee, I. (2013). Serious leisure, life satisfaction, and health of older adults. *Leisure Sciences, 35*(1), 16–32.

Hirao, K., Kobayashi, R., Okishima, K., & Tomokuni, Y. (2012). Flow experience and health related quality of life in community dwelling elderly Japanese. *Nursing and Health Sciences, 14*(1), 52–57.

Johnson, T., Bauler, L., Vos, D., Hifko, A., Garg, P., Ahmed, M., & Raphelson, M. (2020). Virtual reality use for symptom management in palliative care: A pilot study to assess user perceptions. *Journal of Palliative Medicine, 23*(9), 1233–1238. https://doi.org/10.1089/jpm.2019.0411

Jung, M., Jonides, J., Northouse, L., Berman, M. G., Koelling, T. M., & Pressler, S. J. (2017). Randomized crossover study of the natural restorative environment intervention to improve attention and mood in heart failure. *The Journal of Cardiovascular Nursing, 32*(5), 464–479. https://doi.org/10.1097/JCN.0000000000000368

Kaplan, S. (1995). The restorative benefits of nature: Toward an integrative framework. *Journal of Environmental Psychology, 15,* 169–182.

Kaplan, S. (2001). Meditation, restoration and the management of mental fatigue. *Environment and Behaviour, 33,* 480–506.

Kaplan, S., & Berman, M. G. (2010). Directed attention as a common resource for executive functioning and self-regulation. *Perspectives on Psychological Science, 5*(1), 43–57. https://doi.org/10.1177/1745691609356784

Korpela, K. M., Ylén, M., Tyrväinen, L., & Silvennoinen, H. (2008). Determinants of restorative experiences in everyday favourite places. *Health & Place, 14,* 636–652.

Lazarus, R. S., & Folkman, S. (1984). *Stress, appraisal and coping.* Springer.

Moneta, G. B., & Csikszentmihalyi, M. (1996). The effect of perceived challenges and skills on the quality of subjective experience. *Journal of Personality, 64,* 274–310.

Norling, J. C., Sibthorp, J., & Ruddell, E. (2008). Perceived restorativeness for activities scale (PRAS): Development and validation. *Journal of Physical Activity and Health, 5,* 184–195.

Oulasvirta, A., & Blom, J. (2008). Motivations in personalisation behaviour. *Interacting with Computers, 20*(1), 1–16. https://doi.org/10.1016/j.intcom.2007.06.002

Parsons, R., & Hartig, T. (2000). Environmental psychophysiology. In J. T. Cacioppo, L. G. Tassinary, & G. G. Berntson (Eds.), *Handbook of psychophysiology* (pp. 815–846). Cambridge University Press.

Riches, S., Azevedo, L., Bird, L., Pisani, S., & Valmaggia, L. (2021). Virtual reality relaxation for the general population: A systematic review. *Social Psychiatry and Psychiatric Epidemiology, 56*(10), 1707–1727.

Rose, T., Nam, C. S., & Chen, K. B. (2018). Immersion of virtual reality for rehabilitation—review. *Applied Ergonomics, 69,* 153–161. https://doi.org/10.1016/j. apergo.2018.01.009

Ryan, R. M., & Deci, E. L. (2000). Self-determination theory and the facilitation of intrinsic motivation, social development and well-being. *American Psychologist, 55,* 68–78.

Ryan, R. M., & Deci, E. L. (2002). An overview of self-determination theory: An organismic dialectical perspective. In E. L. Deci & R. M. Ryan (Eds.), *Handbook of self-determination research* (pp. 3–33). University of Rochester Press.

Ryan, R. M., & Deci, E. L. (2017). *Self-determination theory: Basic psychological needs in motivation, development, and wellness.* The Guilford Press.

Ryan, R. M., & Deci, E. L. (2022). Self-determination theory. In F. Maggino (Ed.), *Encyclopedia of quality of life and well-being research* (pp. 1–7). Springer Nature Switzerland AG. https://doi.org/10.1007/978-3-319-69909-7_2630-2

Ryan, R. M., Lynch, M. F., Vansteenkiste, M., & Deci, E. L. (2011). Motivation and autonomy in counseling, psychotherapy, and behavior change: A look at theory and practice. *The Counseling Psychologist, 39*(2), 193. https://doi. org/10.1177/0011000009359313

Scates, D., Dickinson, J. I., Sullivan, K., Cline, H., & Balaraman, R. (2020). Using nature-inspired virtual reality as a distraction to reduce stress and pain among cancer patients. *Environment and Behavior, 52*(8), 895–918. https://doi. org/10.1177/0013916520916259

Staats, H., Van Germerden, E., & Hartig, T. (2010). Preference for restorational situations: Interactive effects of attentional state, activity-in-environment and social context. *Leisure Sciences, 32,* 401–417.

Standage, M., & Ryan, R. M. (2020). Self-determination theory in sport and exercise. In G. Tenenbaum & R. C. Eklund (Eds.), *Handbook of sport psychology* (Vol. I, 4th ed., pp. 37–56). John Wiley & Sons, Incorporated.

Trépanier, S.-G., Fernet, C., & Austin, S. (2013). Workplace bullying and psychological health at work: The mediating role of satisfaction of needs for autonomy, competence and relatedness. *Work and Stress, 27*(2), 123–140. https://doi.org/ 10.1080/02678373.2013.782158

Ulrich, R. (1983). Aesthetic and affective response to natural environment. In I. Altman & J. F. Wohlwill (Eds.), *Human behavior and environment: Advances in theory and research* (pp. 85–125). Plenum Press.

Veale, D. (2008). Behavioural activation for depression. *Advances in Psychiatric Treatment, 14,* 29–36.

Villemure, C., & Bushnell, M. C. (2002). Cognitive modulation of pain: How do attention and emotion influence pain processing? *Pain, 95*(3), 195–199. https:// doi.org/10.1016/S0304-3959(02)00007-6

Vohs, K. D., Baumeister, R. F., Schmeichel, B. J., Twenge, J. M., Nelson, N. M., & Tice, D. M. (2008). Making choices impairs subsequent self-control: A limited-resource account of decision making, self-regulation, and active initiative. *Journal of Personality and Social Psychology, 94*(5), 883–898.

Wilkie, S., & Stavridou, A. (2013). Influence of environmental preference and environment type congruence on judgments of restoration potential. *Urban Forestry & Urban Greening, 12*(2), 163–170.

Woo, O. K., Lee, A. M., Ng, R., Eckhoff, D., Lo, R., & Cassinelli, A. (2024). Flourishing-life-of-wish virtual reality relaxation therapy (FLOW-VRT-relaxation) outperforms traditional relaxation therapy in palliative care: Results from a randomized controlled trial. *Frontiers in Virtual Reality, 4*, 1304155.

Section III

Clinical Applications of Virtual Reality in Palliative Care

Based on the understanding of the application of VR in palliative care in Section II, this section adopts the biopsychosocial spiritual model to elaborate in detail the clinical applications of VR interventions. The section begins with Chapter 7, which introduces a range of VR apps that have been investigated under empirical research on using VR interventions for physical and psychological symptom management. Chapter 8 discusses the application of VR interventions for social and spiritual support, while Chapter 9 introduces its application for supporting palliative care providers. Lastly, Chapter 10 provides practical guidance for developing effective VR skills and competencies.

DOI: 10.4324/9781003518327-10

Section III

Clinical Applications of Virtual Reality in Palliative Care

7 Virtual Reality for Physical and Psychological Symptom Management

Introduction

Building on the theoretical foundation in the previous section, this chapter begins to introduce the clinical applications of VR interventions that target the management of physical and psychological symptoms. The VR applications discussed in this chapter have been investigated through preliminary or robust research conducted in clinical or in-home settings involving adult or paediatric populations. The clinical applications of VR introduced in this chapter build upon various treatment modalities such as cognitive behavioural therapy, music therapy, and restoration attention. It is understandable that physical and psychological symptoms intertwine. For ease of reference, the chapter is structured into two sections based on the two chief therapeutic goals, i.e., pain management and wish fulfillment (Table 7.1). The chapter ends with clinical cases that have been elaborated on in Chapter 2, with the use of traditional psychological interventions, but now complemented with VR interventions to address their unmet needs.

Pain Management/Relaxation

Applied VR

1. Overview:
   - A prescription VR-based therapeutics for chronic pain management, which were explicitly developed for medical use and suitable in clinical settings.
2. Targeted Therapeutic Goals:
   - Pain management.

DOI: 10.4324/9781003518327-11

Table 7.1 VR interventions for the management of physical and psychological symptoms

Therapeutic Purposes	VR Interventions
Pain management/ relaxation	AppliedVR Atmosphaeres FLOW-VRT-Relaxation Forest of Serenity Immerxive Sr Nature Trek Nintendo Wii Fit Plus Ocean Rift® Relax VR RelieVRx The Blue
Wish fulfillment	Google Earth VR Oculus library Wishplay

3. Evidence-Based Support:

   • A study conducted by Guenther et al. (2022) reported significant pain reduction during, immediately after, and one hour after using *Applied VR* among patients under palliative care. More than 80% of participants rated the VR experience as "good" or "very good" with the intention of repeated VR sessions.

   • Among a group of adult participants with autoimmune diseases, there was a significant reduction in pain scores after the respiratory biofeedback environment and guided meditation modules of the EaseVR chronic pain platform under *AppliedVR* (Venuturupalli et al., 2019).

4. Virtual Environments and Scenarios:

   • Immersive videos are divided into three categories: journeys (Iceland and London), relaxation (various beaches and secluded places, Tibetan singing bowls, meditation), and animals (Dolphins Healing, Seal Hospital, Wild West, Farm Sanctuary).

5. Customization and Personalization:

   • A variety of immersive 360-degree videos for relaxation, distraction, or escaping reality, and games which allow user selections based on personal preferences and individual needs.

   • Motion sensors allow the user to control their devices via head movements.

6. Remarks:

- *RelieVRx/EaseVRx* will be elaborated on later in this chapter

7. References: https://www.appliedvr.io/

Atmosphaeres

1. Overview:

- 360-degree virtual experiences designed for stress management.

2. Targeted Therapeutic Goals:

- Relaxation in natural experiences.
- Enjoying nature featuring the pure nature sounds and pristine 360° nature visuals.
- Meditation with nature, coaching, and soothing music.
- Travel to places of preference.

3. Virtual Environments and Scenarios:

- Nature experiences such as sunrise serenity.
- Travelling locations such as Croatia, Slovenia, Sexony, Galicia.

4. Customization and Personalization:

- Based on a patient's needs or preferences, therapists can choose from categories including beach, city, and farmland; locations such as Australia and Germany; level of resolution; and type of camera used.

5. Evidence-Based Support:

- The research conducted by Brungardt et al. (2021) investigated the feasibility of a VR-based music therapy intervention, which featured nature-based videos from *Atmosphaeres* with a customized soundtrack with a music therapist for listening during the VR experience. 17 out of 23 patients under palliative care completed the intervention, including 39% during an intensive care unit stay. Participants scored usability above average. 53% chose the highest rating for satisfaction. Most participants spoke favourably of the intervention, describing pleasant emotional and physical responses. The authors concluded that the intervention was feasible, usable, and acceptable for hospitalized palliative care patients.

6. References: https://www.sphaeresvr.com/

FLOW-VRT-Relaxation

1. Overview:

- Flourishing-Life-Of-Wish Virtual Reality Therapy (FLOW-VRT®) is a structured and personalized psychological intervention specially designed for patients in need of palliative care (Woo et al., 2024; Woo & Lee, 2023).
- FLOW-VRT is theoretically founded on flow, self-determination, stress coping, and attention restoration theories.
- FLOW-VRT intends to address patients' needs by alleviating physical and emotional distress, as well as enhancing the quality of end-of-life.
- "FLOW-VRT-Relaxation" refers to a specialized version of FLOW-VRT intervention that focuses on relaxation. It allows patients to choose their preferred VR relaxation experience using freely-available YouTube VR videos.

2. Targeted Therapeutic Goals:

- Physical and psychological symptom management through relaxation
- Wish fulfillment through travelling to a preferred relaxation destination

3. Evidence-Based Support:

- The result from an adequately powered randomized controlled trial (Woo et al., 2024) shows that participants following a FLOW-VRT-Relaxation session presented with significantly lower physical and emotional symptoms when compared with traditional relaxation practice.
- A case report (Woo & Lee, 2023) reported initial evidence supporting its feasibility and therapeutic potential among patients under palliative care for wish fulfillment and symptom management.

4. Virtual Environments and Scenarios:

- Eight videos, which are the eight most popular virtual destinations for relaxation as shown in a result of a survey conducted in a palliative care setting:
- Beach: https://youtu.be/bW9VYhytk-c?si=fx-gwd9jqCYA9Kcl.
- Underwater: https://www.youtube.com/watch?v=bzZEKGRoZwc
- Waterfall: https://youtu.be/yGlgldn5orU?si=BZq0R-2oqY_P8gvD
- Snow mountain: https://youtu.be/kQAlOJhfQ?si=ZqyKWVbE7vroXp74
- Japan Onsen: https://youtu.be/IPgsomPcdBI?si=3xEhJpcTWj9QPjMn
- Japan Sakura: https://youtu.be/Awz-wNJ_bk0?si=oQiyClWEMjYnR8L2
- Forest: https://youtu.be/pXfUhkK_QRQ?si=cnyYSDQvoDrB2dqk
- Cloud/Sky: https://youtu.be/mfQb_b_au2w?si=rCYDI7Xivm9_GCDd

Forest of Serenity

1. Overview:

   - A freely available application that features a 10-minute guide through a forest and waterfall with voice narration.
   - It simulates a secluded clearing and invites users to immerse themselves in its sights and sounds through guided meditation.

2. Targeted Therapeutic Goals:

   - Through guided meditation, the users are prompted to explore the tropical rainforest, aiming to transpose their pain.

3. Evidence-Based Support:

   - In the study of Groninger et al. (2021), participants experienced significant improvement in pain score after either 10-minutes of *Forest of Serenity* or 10 minutes of guided imagery in 2D video; however, the group featuring *Forest of Serenity* experienced a 1.5 unit comparatively greater reduction in pain score compared to guided imagery.

4. Virtual Environments and Scenarios:

   - The virtual environments of the forest with guided meditation.

5. Remarks:

   - *Forest of Serenity* is one of the VR contents under Holosphere VR®.

6. References:

   - https://www.holosphere.co.uk/case-study/forest-of-serenity/
   - https://www.youtube.com/watch?v=LOLfuEUot5s

Immerxive Srl

1. Overview:

   - A VR software consisting of both non-interactive and interactive components.

2. Targeted Therapeutic Goals:

   - To improve the quality of life of cancer patients through pain and anxiety management.

3. Virtual Environments and Scenarios:

   - Non-interactive component includes immersive 360° videos with different natural and relaxing scenarios, such as a seascape, a park, a waterfall, the London Bridge, and a mountain landscape.

- Interactive component includes a basic skill game called "Yuma's World." The user who is surrounded by a calm underwater environment has to reproduce with the controller a displayed "Kanji," that is, a Japanese ideogram that represents concepts like friendship, courage, and strength.

4. Evidence-Based Support:

- Results from the study conducted by Moscato et al. (2021) showed that the symptoms related to pain, depression, anxiety, well-being, and shortness of breath collected immediately after the VR sessions using *Immerxive Srl* at home among the recruited 14 patients showed a significant improvement. The author concluded that VR could represent a suitable complementary tool for psychological treatment in advanced cancer patients assisted at home.

5. Customization and Personalization:

- Users are free to choose the type of content (interactive vs. non-interactive) whenever they use the VR headset.

6. Reference: https://www.immerxive.io/#about

Nature Trek VR

1. Overview:

- An app designed for immersion in nature environments that allows the discovery of different animals, commanding the weather, and taking control of the environment, such as night or day.

2. Targeted Therapeutic Goals:

- Relaxation.

3. Evidence-Based Support:

- In the preliminary study conducted by Austin et al. (2022), participants reported that the VR intervention using *Nature Trek VR* was acceptable and caused few side effects. Participants reported significantly higher levels of presence with the VR compared to the 2D screen. Increased presence was associated with significantly lower pain intensity. The authors supported the idea that both 3D and 2D virtual applications provide pain relief for people receiving palliative care.

4. Virtual Environments and Scenarios:

- Has nine colour-themed environments

- Virtual destinations include tropical beaches, underwater oceans, and the stars.
- Audio visualizations can be activated to create a powerful and emotional affect.

5. Interactive Tools and Activities:

- Snap and hold branches to summon birds and butterflies.
- Utilize the "meditation Lotus" to help control breathing.

6. Customization and Personalization:

- Each environment has been carefully crafted to influence specific emotional states
- Control the weather and time of day.
- Use the "creator orbs" to shape your own world.
- Turn off the music and experience a world filled with the calming, soothing sounds of nature.

7. Reference: https://www.meta.com/experiences/2616537008386430/

Nintendo Wii Fit Plus

1. Overview:

- Wii Fit Plus, an enhanced version of Wii Fit developed by Nintendo EAD, features additional games, activities, and features.

2. Targeted Therapeutic Goals:

- Physical symptom management and health monitoring.

3. Evidence-Based Support:

- A study conducted by Hoffman et al. (2014) supports the feasibility, tolerability, and acceptability of light-intensity exercises using the *Nintendo Wii Fit Plus* (VR approach) for postthoracotomy lung cancer patients. All participants in the study reported mild fatigue levels from weeks 5 through 16, with high levels of confidence in fatigue self-management despite most undergoing adjuvant therapy.

4. Virtual Environments and Scenarios:

- The *Nintendo Wii Fit Plus* provides a virtual environment where the users can view themselves, friends, and even their dog walking on a sunny day next to a stream through a village with happy and familiar faces offering encouragement.

5. Interactive Tools and Activities:

- As users walk in place in their homes, they can see themselves taking a corresponding step in the virtual environment.
- Balance exercises use a gaming format and scoring system as motivation to improve performance. Exercises include downhill skiing, soccer, golf, and video game activities.
- Exercises use competitive and engaging formats, keeping users captivated while they are exercising.
- Walking with the Wii is self-paced (i.e., users can stop instantly, unlike a treadmill).

6. References: https://www.nintendo.com.hk/wiifitplus/wfp_beginner.html (in Chinese)

Ocean Rift®

1. Overview:

- A VR aquatic safari park that explores a vivid underwater world.

2. Targeted Therapeutic Goals:

- Pain and anxiety management.

3. Evidence-Based Support:

- Research conducted by Mohammad and Ahmad (2019) shows that one session of immersive VR using *Ocean Rift*® plus morphine made a significant reduction in pain and anxiety self-reported scores, compared with morphine alone, in patients with breast cancer. The authors conclude that immersive VR is an effective distraction intervention for managing pain and anxiety among breast cancer patients. Using immersive VR as an adjuvant intervention is more effective than morphine alone in relieving pain and anxiety. VR is considered a safe intervention more than pharmacological treatment.

4. Virtual Environments and Scenarios:

- Features 14 habitats, including coral reefs, lagoons, deep ocean, and the Arctic. Users are free to swim around and explore these habitats or teleport between points of interest.
- Several special environments, including beluga whale and great white shark tanks.
- Over 50 animals to discover, including tropical fish, dolphins, sharks, whales, sea lions, manatees, and even prehistoric creatures.

5. Interactive Tools and Activities:

- Users can freely "swim" around and interface with the app using natural hand gestures.

6. References: https://www.meta.com/experiences/2134272053250863/

Relax VR

1. Overview:

- A VR app that allows users to immerse, relax, and escape to locations around the world.

2. Targeted Therapeutic Goals:

- Immersive relaxation and meditation.

3. Evidence-Based Support:

- A feasibility study conducted by Nwosu et al. (2024) reported that all 15 participants recruited from a hospital palliative inpatient unit and a hospice reported positive experiences with no major adverse effects.
- Staff members in palliative care who participated in this study rated VR as helpful and willing to use VR in the future. The reported benefits of VR were its ease of use, the improvements in psychological well-being, and the observed positive short-term effects in participants.

4. Virtual Environments and Scenarios:

- 360-degree video scenes of natural landscapes captured all around the world.
- Spatial 360-degree audio sounds of the beach, ocean, wind, and waves.
- Spatial 360-degree guided meditation recordings in calming voices.

5. Remarks:

- *RelaxVR* has its own device, which is no longer supported by Oculus.

6. References: https://www.relaxvr.co/

RelieVRx

1. Overview:

- *RelieVRx* is a prescription-use immersive VR system intended to provide adjunctive treatment based on cognitive behavioural therapy and other evidence-based behavioural methods for adult patients diagnosed with chronic lower back pain.

- The first adjunctive VR treatment at home for chronic lower back pain authorized by the U.S. Food and Drug Administration.
- Consists of mindful escape, pain education, diaphragmatic breathing, and relaxation modules.

2. Targeted Therapeutic Goals:

- For in-home pain management in patients with chronic lower back pain.

3. Evidence-Based Support:

- In the study of Garcia et al. (2021), *EaseVRx* was found to have high user satisfaction and symptom reduction for average pain intensity and pain-related interference with activity, mood, and stress when compared to a 2D nature content delivered in a VR headset.
- Maddox et al. (2023) reported that *RelieVRx* imparts clinically meaningful improvements above a strong, active control comparison on pain intensity and pain interference in clinically severe and diverse adults with chronic low back pain.

4. Virtual Environments and Scenarios:

- Serene nature landscapes, tranquil beaches, or peaceful gardens.

5. Practical Considerations:

- *RelieVRx* requires VR headsets and compatible hardware for optimal use.
- The app offers technical support and training resources to assist therapists in implementing and utilizing the application.

6. Remarks:

- Formerly known as *EaseVRx*.
- *RelieVRx* is under *AppliedVR*.

7. Reference: https://www.relievrx.com/

The Blu

1. Overview:

- A VR series that allows users to experience the ocean through different habitats.

2. Targeted Therapeutic Goals:

- To provide a virtual experience in various sea habitats for the benefits of pain management or positive engagement.

3. Evidence-Based Support:

   • Research from Kelleher et al. (2022) supports the feasibility, acceptability, and safety of *VR Blue* for advanced colorectal cancer patients. Participants showed significant pre-post improvement in pain and pain-related symptoms, shedding light on the potential feasibility of VR interventions in this population.

4. Virtual Environments and Scenarios:

   • The app has three virtual environments:

     1. Whale Encounter: An undersea encounter with a blue whale, the largest species on earth.
     2. Reef Migration: A witness of an undersea migration on the edge of a coral reef.
     3. Luminous Abyss: A venture into the deepest region of the ocean to discover the iridescent abyss.

5. Interactive Tools and Activities:

   • *VR Blue* offers six degrees of freedom, which means that not only can the users turn their head to look in any direction, but they can also shift their location, for example, looking behind a rock, bending down in order to closer inspect an underwater plant, or ducking to avoid an intrusive fish.
   • Users may slow time and capture pictures in Inspector Mode and return to a meditative version of each location in Ambient Mode.

6. References: https://wevr.com/theblu

Wish Fulfillment

Google Earth VR

1. Overview:

   • *Google Earth VR* utilizes satellite imagery, 3D terrain data, and Street View imagery from Google Maps, allowing users to navigate and explore various locations worldwide, including landmarks, cities, and natural wonders.

2. Targeted Therapeutic Goals:

   • To fulfill the wishes of travelling to a place that is meaningful to an individual patient, such as a childhood village, the streets of Tokyo, the Grand Canyon, or the Eiffel Tower.

3. Evidence-Based Support:

   • A preliminary study conducted by Niki et al. (2019) revealed significant improvement in pain, fatigue, drowsiness, breathlessness, depression, and anxiety among 20 patients from palliative care wards after a 30-minute session of using the *Google Earth VR* app.

4. Virtual Environments and Scenarios:

- It offers the ability to fly above cities, zoom in to street-level views, and explore underwater environments.

5. Practical Considerations:

- *Google Earth VR* is supported by SteamVR or Oculus PC.

6. Reference: https://store.steampowered.com/app/348250/Google_Earth_VR/?l=tchinese

Oculus Library

1. Overview:

- A collection of applications, games, and experiences available on the Oculus VR platform developed by Meta.

2. Targeted Therapeutic Goals:

- To meet various needs of individual patients.

3. Evidence-Based Support:

- In the pilot study of Johnson et al. (2020), 12 adult patients with life-limiting illnesses chose their specific VR application(s) based on a "menu" of nine options that were pre-selected by the research team with a focus on low-cost, easy-to-learn applications. All of these applications include auditory and visual components, with visual components ranging from photorealistic still images to animated videos. The intervention lasted for 30 minutes. Participants found the VR experience enjoyable and useful, and the intervention was overall well-tolerated.

4. Virtual Environments and Scenarios:

- 360 Photos: https://www.meta.com/experiences/922519877806282/
- Meditation: https://www.meta.com/experiences/3385318684883998/
- Apollo 11: https://www.meta.com/experiences/pcvr/1943333329057022/
- Bait!: https://www.meta.com/experiences/2082595615120854/#?
- Feel: The Must of the Sea: https://ilovethesea.es/feel/
- Bear Island: https://www.meta.com/experiences/pcvr/1228652173894654/

- theBlu: https://www.meta.com/experiences/pcvr/984294025016007/
- Coaster: https://www.meta.com/experiences/2299465166734471/
- Hello Mars: https://www.meta.com/experiences/1263460633768255/

Wishplay

1. Overview:
   - A website with a collection of VR videos that offers users the opportunity to explore destinations that hold special significance to them.

2. Targeted Therapeutic Goals:
   - To help combat the boredom and fatigue of patients in palliative and long-term care.
   - To grant wishes to those who are unable to play in the real world.

3. Evidence-Based Support:
   - With the founder's support, *Wishplay* app was reportedly used by a young girl in paediatric palliative care (Weingarten et al., 2020). The authors conclude the significant potential for VR in paediatric palliative care.

4. Virtual Environments and Scenarios:
   - Ranging from fantastical landscapes to engaging in thrilling adventures. Examples include strolling through the forest and enjoying the aurora borealis.

5. References:
   - www.wishplay.ca
   - https://www.youtube.com/channel/UCp7nJA57g40rWyerrX1WaRw

Case Studies

This section presents clinical case studies that demonstrate the integration of traditional psychological interventions with VR technologies which appears to address patients' unmet needs.

Mr. Alpha

Mr. Alpha, a 68-year-old man diagnosed with stage IV lung cancer, currently stays at a residential care home for older adults. His primary concern is shortness of breath, which significantly impacts his quality of life. The difficulty in breathing not only causes physical discomfort but also leads to his fear that he is losing his breath. He also expresses feelings of inadequacy and helplessness in coping with the breathing difficulty. He expressed his wish to travel in natural environments, such as beaches and mountains, for a more peaceful mind.

Elaborated on in Chapter 2, cognitive-behavioural therapy can be applied to help Mr. Alpha through psychoeducation, cognitive processing, and breathing exercises. Despite the therapeutic benefits of cognitive-behavioural therapy, Mr. Alpha's wish of travelling to the natural environment remains unfulfilled. Capitalizing on the sense of presence and immersion, as elaborated on in Chapters 4 and 6, VR technology may help him virtually travel to beaches or mountains with the sense of "being there." One VR psychological intervention, FLOW-VRT-Relaxation (Woo et al., 2024), can be conducted to fulfill Mr. Alpha's wishes while performing relaxation exercises. The procedure, according to the research protocol of Woo et al. (2024), is as follows.

1. Conduct need assessment
2. Present the list of popular VR content for relaxation among palliative care patients, i.e., the scenery of mountain, lake, beach, forest, Japan Onsen, Sakura, sky, and underwater world, and ask the patient to choose the preferred VR content
3. Conduct the VR experience (10 minutes), with video retrieved from *YouTube VR* app
4. Coach the relaxation during a VR experience

Mrs. Delta

Mrs. Delta, a 78-year-old woman, is currently facing the challenges of metastatic cancer and cord compression. These conditions have left her bedbound, requiring specialized care in a rehabilitation hospital. She presents with unresolved pain and emotional distress. When adjusting to tetraplegia, she expresses a sense of meaninglessness and a passive death wish. Mrs. Delta feels frustrated and saddened by her physical limitations, which have impacted her ability to engage in activities she once enjoyed. She is concerned about her ability to fulfill her mother's role and struggles with feelings of worthlessness. She also expressed her wish to see the aurora borealis, which has been the dream of her life.

Meaning-based interventions, as elaborated on in Chapter 2, have been one of the traditional approaches supporting Mrs. Delta's psychological needs. She can explore with the therapist her personal meaning and purpose in life despite the physical constraints and terminal illnesses. Although the meaning-based interventions bring along certain therapeutic benefits, her wish to see the aurora borealis remains unfulfilled. VR may then intervene to help wish fulfillment in a virtual but immersive way. *YouTube VR* apps provide various high-quality VR videos of aurora borealis, as one of the chosen videos in the study of Woo et al. (2024). Another VR app is *Google Earth VR*, which utilizes satellite imagery from Google Maps (Niki et al., 2019) that allows Mrs. Delta to explore the North Pole region.

Conclusions

The diverse VR interventions examined in this chapter highlight the tremendous potential of this technology to enhance the management of physical and psychological symptoms in palliative care. VR technology appears to be a therapeutic tool that has been supported by empirical research on its pain management, relaxation, and wish fulfillment. As regulatory bodies like the U.S. Food and Drug Administration begin to approve VR systems for prescription use, the integration of these cutting-edge interventions into standard palliative care practices appears to be increasingly feasible. The advancement of VR technology is foreseeable in the near future, which aims to empower patients to take an active and self-determined role during their rehabilitation journey at the end-of-life stage.

References

Austin, P. D., Siddall, P. J., & Lovell, M. R. (2022). Feasibility and acceptability of virtual reality for cancer pain in people receiving palliative care: A randomised cross-over study. *Supportive Care in Cancer: Official Journal of the Multinational Association of Supportive Care in Cancer*, 30(5), 3995–4005. https://doi.org/10.1007/s00520-022-06824-x

Brungardt, A., Wibben, A., Tompkins, A. F., Shanbhag, P., Coats, H., LaGasse, A. B., Boeldt, D., Youngwerth, J., Kutner, J. S., & Lum, H. D. (2021). Virtual reality-based music therapy in palliative care: A pilot implementation trial. *Journal of Palliative Medicine*, 24(5), 736–742.

Garcia, L. M., Birckhead, B. J., Krishnamurthy, P., Sackman, J., Mackey, I. G., Louis, R. G., Salmasi, V., Maddox, T., & Darnall, B. D. (2021). An 8-week self-administered at-home behavioral skills-based virtual reality program for chronic low back pain: Double-blind, randomized, placebo-controlled trial conducted during COVID–19. *Journal of Medical Internet Research*, 23(2), e26292. https://doi.org/10.2196/26292

Groninger, H., Stewart, D., Fisher, J. M., Tefera, E., Cowgill, J., & Mete, M. (2021). Virtual reality for pain management in advanced heart failure: A randomized controlled study. *Palliative Medicine*, 35(10), 2008–2016. https://doi.org/10.1177/02692163211041273

Guenther, M., Görlich, D., Bernhardt, F., Pogatzki-Zahn, E., Dasch, B., Krueger, J., & Lenz, P. (2022). Virtual reality reduces pain in palliative care–a feasibility trial. *BMC Palliative Care, 21*(1), 169.

Hoffman, A. J., Brintnall, R. A., Brown, J. K., Von Eye, A., Jones, L. W., Alderink, G., Ritz-Holland, D., Enter, M., Patzelt, L. H., & VanOtteren, G. M. (2014). Virtual reality bringing a new reality to postthoracotomy lung cancer patients via a home-based exercise intervention targeting fatigue while undergoing adjuvant treatment. *Cancer Nursing, 37*(1), 23–33.

Johnson, T., Bauler, L., Vos, D., Hifko, A., Garg, P., Ahmed, M., & Raphelson, M. (2020). Virtual reality use for symptom management in palliative care: A pilot study to assess user perceptions. *Journal of Palliative Medicine, 23*(9), 1233–1238.

Kelleher, S. A., Fisher, H. M., Winger, J. G., Miller, S. N., Amaden, G. H., Somers, T. J., Colloca, L., Uronis, H. E., & Keefe, F. J. (2022). Virtual reality for improving pain and pain-related symptoms in patients with advanced stage colorectal cancer: A pilot trial to test feasibility and acceptability. *Palliative & Supportive Care, 20*(4), 471–481.

Maddox, T., Oldstone, L., Sparks, C. Y., Sackman, J., Oyao, A., Garcia, L., Maddox, R. U., Ffrench, K., Garcia, H., Adair, T., Irvin, A., Maislin, D., Keenan, B., Bonakdar, R., & Darnall, B. D. (2023). In-home virtual reality program for chronic lower back pain: A randomized Sham-controlled effectiveness trial in a clinically severe and diverse sample. *Mayo Clinic Proceedings: Digital Health, 1*(4), 563–573. https://doi.org/10.1016/j.mcpdig.2023.09.003

Mohammad, E. B., & Ahmad, M. (2019). Virtual reality as a distraction technique for pain and anxiety among patients with breast cancer: A randomized control trial. *Palliative & Supportive Care, 17*(1), 29–34.

Moscato, S., Sichi, V., Giannelli, A., Palumbo, P., Ostan, R., & Chiari, L. (2021). Virtual reality in home palliative care: Brief report on the effect on cancer-related symptomatology. *Frontiers in Psychology, 12,* 709154.

Niki, K., Okamoto, Y., Maeda, I., Mori, I., Ishii, R., Matsuda, Y., Takagi, T., & Uejima, E. (2019). A novel palliative care approach using virtual reality for improving various symptoms of terminal cancer patients: A preliminary prospective, multicenter study. *Journal of Palliative Medicine, 22*(6), 702–707.

Nwosu, A. C., Mills, M., Roughneen, S., Stanley, S., Chapman, L., & Mason, S. R. (2024). Virtual reality in specialist palliative care: A feasibility study to enable clinical practice adoption. *BMJ Supportive & Palliative Care, 14*(1), 47–51. https://doi.org/10.1136/bmjspcare-2020-002327

Venuturupalli, R. S., Chu, T., Vicari, M., Kumar, A., Fortune, N., & Spielberg, B. (2019). Virtual reality–based biofeedback and guided meditation in rheumatology: A pilot study. *ACR Open Rheumatology, 1*(10), 667–675.

Weingarten, K., Macapagal, F., & Parker, D. (2020). Virtual reality: Endless potential in pediatric palliative care: A case report. *Journal of Palliative Medicine, 23*(1), 147–149.

Woo, O. K. L., & Lee, A. M. (2023). Case report: Therapeutic potential of flourishing-life-of-wish virtual reality therapy on relaxation (FLOW-VRT-relaxation)— a novel personalized relaxation in palliative care. *Frontiers in Digital Health, 5.* https://doi.org/10.3389/fdgth.2023.1228781

Woo, O. K. L., Lee, A. M., Ng, R., Eckhoff, D., Lo, R., & Cassinelli, A. (2024). Flourishing-life-of-wish virtual reality relaxation therapy (FLOW-VRT-relaxation) outperforms traditional relaxation therapy in palliative care: Results from a randomized controlled trial. *Frontiers in Virtual Reality, 4,* 1304155. https://doi.org/10.3389/frvir.2023.1304155

8 Virtual Reality for Social and Spiritual Support

Introduction

In addition to addressing physical and psychological needs, there is empirical evidence supporting the use of VR technology in fulfilling the social and spiritual needs of patients as well. The chapter is structured into two sections introducing VR interventions on facilitating social and spiritual support (Table 8.1). It ends with clinical cases that had been elaborated in Chapter 2 with the use of traditional psychological interventions, now complemented with VR interventions to address the unmet social and spiritual needs of individual patients.

Social Support Interventions

The Use of VR Camera

1. Overview:

   - To produce a personalized VR video by family members or carers for hospitalized patients.

2. Targeted Therapeutic Goals:

   - To reduce feelings of loneliness among patients who need long-term hospitalization that may affect the quality of end-of-life.

3. Evidence-Based Support:

   - In the study of Mukai et al. (2023), family members of the patients in hospital-based palliative care were asked to take videos of themselves at home and other familiar places where the patients wished to visit using a VR camera. The study results attained by text mining suggest the promising potential of VR in reducing the pain of hospitalization by feeling safe and secure with family members, regaining daily life, and providing an immersive feeling of being in the same space with family.

DOI: 10.4324/9781003518327-12

Table 8.1 VR interventions for social and spiritual support

Therapeutic Purposes	VR Interventions
Social Support	The use of VR camera Unity Second Life® The livestreaming function
Spiritual Support	VoicingHan A VR-based life review therapy system
Other Support	VR Stimulation for Advance Care Planning

Unity

1. Overview:

   • A game engine and development platform that helps create VR experiences.

2. Targeted Therapeutic Goals:

   • To facilitate active rehabilitation.

3. Evidence-Based Support:

   • A feasibility study conducted by Ando et al. (2020) recruited five cancer patients for the VR cancer peer support program. The program had five kinds of virtual worlds (i.e., seashore, football stadium, sports gym, boxing ring, and the woods) where the virtual exercise trainer appeared once every 20 minutes. An avatar was created as a proxy for the participant. The virtual trainer instructed and performed exercise simultaneously for about 10 minutes and then disappeared during the 10-minute interval. The authors concluded that the VR peer training program is considered useful for reducing physical laziness and encouraging participants to maintain exercise habits after completion.

4. References: https://unity.com/cn

Second Life®

1. Overview:

   • A life-simulation network that allows users to create and manage the lives of avatars they create in an advanced social setting with other online "residents."

2. Targeted Therapeutic Goals:

- Social support for bereavement.

3. Evidence-Based Support:

- In a controlled study conducted by Knowles et al. (2017), 30 widow(er)s either participated in an 8-week VR support group using *Second Life®* or accessed a grief education website.
- Both groups showed significant improvements in grief severity, grief cognitions, yearning, loneliness, perceived stress, and global sleep quality across study time points. However, only widow(er)s in the VR support group showed a significant improvement in depression over time.
- The author concludes the feasibility, acceptability, and preliminary efficacy of an accessible and low-cost online support format for widow(er)s.

4. Virtual Environments and Scenarios:

- Virtual worlds have two advantages over existing online support programme that facilitate interpersonal relationships and emotional support (Gorini et al., 2008; Green-Hamann et al., 2011). First, the virtual world allows users to communicate with each other in real-time. Second, users are embodied as avatars and interact with their surroundings and other users' avatars.

5. Remarks:

- *Second Life®* is a free virtual world software program.

6. References: https://secondlife.com/

The Livestreaming Function

1. Overview:

- Livestreaming function of VR allows users to connect with others in a shared virtual space, enabling live participation in events, training sessions, or support groups, regardless of their physical location.

2. Targeted Therapeutic Goals:

- To virtually participate in a self-selected event that happens in real-time to facilitate a sense of social presence, i.e., the sense of being with others in a virtual environment, with the use of a VR camera.

3. Evidence-Based Support:

- Emerging studies have investigated the use of the livestreaming function of VR in medical fields such as surgery (Gandsas et al., 2023; Long et al., 2023).
- To my knowledge, there have been no studies validating the use of livestreaming function of VR technology in a palliative care setting. However, its special function reveals its potential in catering to the social needs of patients under palliative care.

Spiritual Support Interventions

VoicingHan

1. Overview:

- An avatar-mediated life-review project designed for cancer patients in palliative care settings.

2. Targeted Therapeutic Goals:

- Life review interventions.

3. Evidence-Based Support:

- In a study conducted by Ryu and Price (2022), 12 patients receiving outpatient palliative care had a 30–40-minute sessions of spontaneously engaged avatar life-review, starting from childhood to the current developmental stage. The storytelling performances were recorded via avatar video format and distributed to the participants for their review, sharing, and legacy document. Post-survey found all patients agreed or strongly agreed they would participate again, recommend it to others, and found the experience beneficial. After one month, palliative care scores were either unchanged or improved in 80% of patients. The authors concluded that the avatar-facilitated life review was feasible with a high rate of adherence, completion, and acceptability by patients.

A VR-Based Life-Review Therapy System

1. Overview:

- A VR-based life-review therapy system that facilitates life-review therapy using customized photos and videos from patients in a virtual space resonant with personal and historical memory.

2. Targeted Therapeutic Goals:

   - To allow patients to reminisce about their past with the therapist and create a meaningful narrative about their lives.

3. Evidence-Based Support:

   - The study conducted by Ng et al. (2024) details the participatory design of the systems. The evaluation of the qualitative feedback about the system concluded that it was a feasible and effective intervention.

4. Virtual Environments and Scenarios:

   - There are three virtual environments:

     1. A relaxing and neutral pre-therapy space, which is an empty room with relaxation music, a mountain view, and a tree is intended to prepare users for life review interventions.
     2. The therapy space is modelled after a traditional Hong Kong-style Tong Lau apartment reminiscent of 1960s and 1970s Hong Kong. Features include a television playing historical TVB new footage from Hong Kong, a record player playing Cantonese pop music from the 1960s, and nostalgic décor, all of which aim to encourage the users to reminisce about their past. In the apartment, there are patients' own photographs and videos, which act as a catalyst for the patient to speak about their past.
     3. The post-therapy nature space, i.e., a beach, in which the patient can relax and have a debrief with the therapist on the life review intervention.

5. Interactive Tools and Activities:

   - There are two interactive elements: the photo albums which have content from the patient's own lives which the therapist had toggle through, the mahjong table where patients can play mahjong.

6. Integration with Traditional Therapies:

   - The VR life review therapy system is an adaptation of traditional life review therapy, which allows patients' family members, who may not be able to enter palliative care wards, to collaborate on this process virtually.

7. Remarks:

   - The system requires at least two Meta Quest II VR headsets and a good internet connection. It also requires some extra space in the hospital for the therapist to be able to move around.

Other Support Interventions

A Stimulation for Advance Care Planning

1. Overview:

   - A 6-minute educational VR video for advance care planning with the first-person perspective of a patient with COPD to allow participants to immerse themselves in the complete clinical process of typical end-of-life care.

2. Targeted Goals:

   - To facilitate decisions related to advance care planning.

3. Evidence-Based Support:

   - Hsieh (2020) studied the change in participants' preference and certainty regarding end-of-life decisions after using a VR video before advance care planning.
   - The author reported that after viewing the VR video, preference for not using cardiopulmonary resuscitation, life-sustaining treatment, antibiotics, blood transfusion, and artificial nutrition and hydration increased significantly in the VR intervention group. Uncertainty regarding the five medical options mentioned previously significantly decreased. The intervention was generally recognized by participants for its help in making decisions. The decrease in the number of participants who could not make decisions indicates that the VR video may be helpful for users in making end-of-life decisions.
   - The author concluded that the VR video helped equip users with a better understanding of medical scenarios and that it is a good decision tool for advance care planning.

Case Studies

This section presents clinical case studies that demonstrate the integration of traditional psychological interventions with VR technologies which appears to address patients' unmet needs.

Mrs. Beta

Mrs. Beta, a 72-year-old woman diagnosed with advanced breast cancer, currently stays at a residential care home for older adults. She presents with significant anxiety related to her illness. As a mother, she feels inadequate and sad about being unable to attend her daughter's upcoming wedding. She feels defeated every time when she tries to get rid of her worrying thoughts.

Traditional approaches, such as mindfulness-based interventions as elaborated on in Chapter 2, can help Mrs. Beta cope with future-oriented and anxious thinking. However, her wish to attend her daughter's upcoming wedding remains unattainable. To maximize the sense of involvement in the wedding, VR technology can intervene to facilitate the sense of social presence, as elaborated on in Chapter 4. One approach is to use the recording function of the VR camera, as reported in Mukai et al. (2023). Family members of the patients can be invited to take the VR videos of the wedding ceremonies. It can also be achieved through the trial use of livestreaming function, which allows Mrs. Beta to "participate" virtually in real-time through the VR camera (which is placed in the wedding venue) and the VR headset (which is administered in the hospital setting).

Mrs. Charlie

Mrs. Charlie, a 68-year-old woman with advanced pancreatic cancer, now stays in an isolated room of a residential unit for older adults for infection control. Given the restricted visiting hours, she feels lonely and disconnected from her usual social support networks. She longs for companionship and emotional support. She wishes to reunite with her husband and have a heartfelt dinner with children at her own home.

Similar to Mrs. Beta, Mrs. Charlie has unfulfilled wishes due to physical constraints. Traditional social support interventions can help Mrs. Charlie to cope emotionally with the end-of-life challenge, as elaborated on in Chapter 2. Through visits from healthcare professionals, friends, family members, or volunteers, meaningful and social activities can be facilitated. Social support groups can also play a role. Despite the traditional approach, her wish of having a heartfelt dinner with children at home has yet been fulfilled. Capitalizing on the advanced VR technology, the virtual travel to home may partly facilitate the heartfelt dinner. It can be achieved through VR video filming similar to the intervention delivered to Mrs. Beta. One approach is to invite family members to use the recording function of the VR camera (Mukai et al., 2023) and take the VR videos at home. Another approach can be the trial use of livestreaming function, which allows Mrs. Charlie to view the real-time 360-degree video from the VR camera (which is placed at home) using a VR headset (which is administered in the hospital setting).

Mrs. Echo

Mrs. Echo is an 85-year-old woman with end-stage renal disease. She is bored at hostel and eager to share her personal views and experiences. Her illness and the resulting physical restrictions have limited her activities, leading to a sense of purposelessness in her daily life. Mrs. Echo yearns to connect with others and share her life experiences.

Traditional reminiscence therapy, as elaborated on in Chapter 2, can help Mrs. Echo to review and reintegrate past experiences using prompts or cues such as photos, videos, music, or objects. Dignity therapy can help him create a legacy document that captures significant past events. Taking advantage of the sense of presence, VR technology allows an immersive life review experience. *VoicingHan*, as an avatar-facilitated life review using synchronized, personalized avatars in VR, may be applied to Mrs. Echo. The personalized element includes the use of an avatar storytelling platform with five environmental options to be chosen by Mrs. Echo (beach, mountain, city, living room, and empty space). VR interventions also serve as a helpful alternative to provide Mrs. Echo with a variety of virtual activities, ranging from fantastical landscapes to engaging in thrilling adventures, through the use of Wishplay (see Chapter 7), which is specially designed to help combat the boredom of patients in palliative and long-term care.

Conclusions

This chapter introduces VR interventions that aim to address the social and spiritual needs of patients. The case studies presented illustrate how VR can be integrated into palliative care. As patients under palliative care are often constrained by physical fragility, the continued advancement and adoption of these VR-based interventions appear to be crucial to address patient's social or spiritual needs that may not be well addressed by traditional practices.

References

Ando, M., Sumitani, M., Sakamura, M., Noguchi, T., Oki, R., Abe, H., Inoue, R., Tsuchida, R., & Uchida, K. (2020). Tele virtual reality-based peer support programme for cancer patients: A preliminary feasibility and acceptability study. *British Journal of Cancer Research, 3*(4), 443–448.

Gandsas, A., Dorey, T., & Park, A. (2023). Immersive live streaming of surgery using 360-degree video to head-mounted virtual reality devices: A new paradigm in surgical education. *Surgical Innovation, 30*(4), 486–492. https://doi.org/10.1177/15533506231165828

Gorini, A., Gaggioli, A., Vigna, C., & Riva, G. (2008). A second life for eHealth: Prospects for the use of 3-D virtual worlds in clinical psychology. *Journal of Medical Internet Research, 10*(3), e21. http://dx.doi.org/10.2196/jmir.1029

Green-Hamann, S., Campbell Eichhorn, K., & Sherblom, J. C. (2011). An exploration of why people participate in second life social support groups. *Journal of Computer-Mediated Communication, 16*(4), 465e491. http://dx.doi.org/10.1111/j.1083-6101.2011.01543.x

Hsieh, W. T. (2020). Virtual reality video promotes effectiveness in advance care planning. *BMC Palliative Care, 19*, 1–10.

Knowles, L. M., Stelzer, E. M., Jovel, K. S., & O'Connor, M. F. (2017). A pilot study of virtual support for grief: Feasibility, acceptability, and preliminary outcomes. *Computers in Human Behavior, 73*, 650–658.

Long, A. S., Almeida, M. N., Chong, L., & Prsic, A. (2023). Live virtual surgery and virtual reality in surgery: Potential applications in hand surgery education. *The Journal of Hand Surgery (American Edition), 48*(5), 499–505. https://doi.org/10.1016/j.jhsa.2023.01.004

Mukai, T., Tsukiyama, Y., Yamada, S., Nishikawa, A., Hayami, S., Noguchi, R., Yoshida, J., Kashiwada, M., Ohta, S., Shimokawa, T., & Yamaue, H. (2023). Virtual reality images of the home are useful for patients with hospital-based palliative care: Prospective observational study with analysis by text mining. *Palliative Medicine Reports, 4*(1), 214–219. https://doi.org/10.1089/pmr.2023.0017

Ng, R., Woo, O. K. L., Eckhoff, D., Zhu, M., Lee, A. M., & Cassinelli, A. (2024). Participatory design of a virtual reality life review therapy system for palliative care. *Frontiers in Virtual Reality, 5*. https://doi.org/10.3389/frvir.2024.1304615

Ryu, S., & Price, S. K. (2022). Embodied storytelling and meaning-making at the end of life: VoicingHan avatar life-review for palliative care in cancer patients. *Arts & Health, 14*(3), 326–340.

9 Virtual Reality for Supporting Palliative Care Providers

Introduction

As the complexities of palliative care continue to evolve, innovative interventions are essential not only for patients and their families but also for palliative care providers striving to deliver compassionate care. The current chapter proceeds to introduce VR interventions that provide relevant support for professionals involved in palliative care. It introduces a range of VR-based applications designed to improve the skills and experiences of palliative care providers, including medical students, nurses, and palliative care specialists. The applications include simulations to enhance communication when breaking bad news, peer storytelling sessions to support adaptive grief, simulated palliative and end-of-life care conferences, immersive resources for facilitating medical students' understanding of palliative care, and emotional support for palliative care providers.

Second Life®

1. Overview:
   - A life-simulation network that allows users to create and manage the lives of avatars they create in an advanced social setting with other online "residents."

2. Targeted Goals:
   - Effective communication of medical students when breaking bad news (Andrade et al., 2010).
   - Peer storytelling sessions to support oncology nurses dealing with grief (Rice et al., 2014).
   - Simulated palliative and end-of-life care conferences (Sanborn et al., 2019).
   - Promotion of interprofessional collaboration among healthcare students with team building activities, team meetings with standardized patient and family, and team debriefing about the experience (Lee et al., 2020).

DOI: 10.4324/9781003518327-13

3. Evidence-Based Support:

- In the study of Andrade et al. (2010) on avatar-mediated training in the delivery of bad news in a virtual world, all participants who were medical trainees considered the experience positive and commended such a novel approach. Participants appraised the training as an excellent approach to learning how to deliver bad news but suggested that it could not substitute for interactions with patients in real life. However, the self-efficacy of participants improved, indicating a variable educational approach for skill training in delivering bad news.

- Rice et al. (2014) suggests a potential benefit of using peer storytelling sessions in *Second Life®* to facilitate oncology nurses' grief resolution. It provides a non-threatening venue for participating nurses to share their innermost feelings and accrue their own inventory of stories.

- Sanborn et al. (2019), in a short report, proposed a 6-week learning activity using an online VR environment through *Second Life®* to advance interprofessional education with a sample of undergraduate and graduate health professions learners through a simulated palliative and end-of-life care conference. The authors reported that VR engaged learners in realistic scenarios in a safe environment free from the risk of harm to patients and families, allowing small groups of learners to meet synchronously online and providing an alternative to face-to-face synchronous scheduling of multiple health professions disciplines, thus reducing strain on program budgets and scheduling logistics.

- Lee et al. (2020) investigated the use of a virtual world educational environment for interprofessional health professions students learning about palliative care. The study results showed that the educational experience was acceptable to participants, with an improvement in attitudes toward interprofessional education and interprofessional teamwork after a single virtual world educational session, based on both quantitative and qualitative results.

4. Virtual Environments and Scenarios:

- Virtual worlds have two advantages over existing online support programme that facilitate interpersonal relationships and emotional support (Gorini et al., 2008; Green-Hamann et al., 2011). First, the virtual world allows users to communicate with each other in real-time. Second, users are embodied as avatars and interact with their surroundings and other users' avatars.

5. Remarks:

- *Second Life®* is a free virtual world software program.

6. References: https://secondlife.com/

VR Stimulation for Medical Teaching

1. Overview:

   - A 27-minute VR lecture on nausea and vomiting management in palliative care and oncology settings and a VR experience of radiotherapy from a patient's viewpoint.

2. Targeted Goals:

   - Using immersive VR to enhance medical students' perceptions of palliative care.

3. Evidence-Based Support:

   - Taubert et al. (2019) studied the use of VR stimulation for medical teaching. Of the 72 medical students who participated, 70 found the experience comfortable, with two students stating they felt the experience uncomfortable. Numerical scoring on the ability to concentrate in VR from 0 to 10 (0=worst, 10=best) scored an average of 8. When asked whether this format suited their learning style, the average score was 8. More than 97% of students stated that they would recommend this form of learning to a colleague. The authors concluded that the VR immersive environments in medical teaching in palliative care and oncology have been well received by medical students.

4. References:

   - VR lecture: https://www.youtube.com/watch?v=F3DEnWvF4Lk&t=1s&ab_channel=Velindrecc
   - VR experience of radiotherapy: https://www.youtube.com/watch?v=7WwNvXjVHQ8&ab_channel=Velindrecc

TRIPP

1. Overview:

   - *TRIPP* is an app designed to help manage emotional well-being through VR immersion.

2. Targeted Goals:

   - To improve the emotional well-being of palliative care providers.

3. Evidence-Based Support:

   - Mercante et al. (2024) investigated the feasibility, safety, and efficacy of a VR intervention using *TRIPP* in relieving the psychological distress of palliative care staff working in a paediatric hospice.

- The VR intervention is a 10-minute session of an English demo version of the *TRIPP* software, created to induce relaxation. It offered a fully immersive meditation experience through soothing voice-guiding subjects in their interactions with virtual worlds and breathing exercises.
- The result showed that participants were calmer, more relaxed, and feeling safer after the VR intervention. Tension and restlessness were reduced. The mean mood score significantly improved. All the participants found the VR a pleasant experience.

4. References: https://www.tripp.com/

Conclusions

This chapter highlights the immense potential of VR interventions to support and empower palliative care providers in their challenging and demanding roles. As the demand for high-quality palliative care continues to grow, the continued development of VR-based interventions will be crucial in equipping and empowering the palliative care workforce with the adequate knowledge, skills, emotional support, and resilience necessary to deliver compassionate and person-centred care.

References

Andrade, A. D., Bagri, A., Zaw, K., Roos, B. A., & Ruiz, J. G. (2010). Avatar-mediated training in the delivery of bad news in a virtual world. *Journal of Palliative Medicine*, *13*(12), 1415–1419.

Gorini, A., Gaggioli, A., Vigna, C., & Riva, G. (2008). A second life for eHealth: Prospects for the use of 3-D virtual worlds in clinical psychology. *Journal of Medical Internet Research*, *10*(3), e21. http://dx.doi.org/10.2196/jmir.1029

Green-Hamann, S., Campbell Eichhorn, K., & Sherblom, J. C. (2011). An exploration of why people participate in second life social support groups. *Journal of Computer-Mediated Communication*, *16*(4), 465–491. http://dx.doi.org/10.1111/j.1083-6101.2011.01543.x

Lee, A. L., DeBest, M., Koeniger-Donohue, R., Strowman, S. R., & Mitchell, S. E. (2020). The feasibility and acceptability of using virtual world technology for interprofessional education in palliative care: A mixed methods study. *Journal of Interprofessional Care*, *34*(4), 461–471. https://doi.org/10.1080/13561820.2019.1643832

Mercante, A., Zanin, A., Vecchi, L., De Tommasi, V., & Benini, F. (2024). Virtual reality intervention as support to paediatric palliative care providers: A pilot study. *Acta Paediatrica*, *113*(4), 833–834. https://doi.org/10.1111/apa.17099

Rice, K. L., Bennett, M. J., & Billingsley, L. (2014). Using second life to facilitate peer storytelling for grieving oncology nurses. *Ochsner Journal*, *14*(4), 551–562.

Sanborn, H., Cole, J., Kennedy, T., & Saewert, K. J. (2019). Practicing interprofessional communication competencies with health profession learners in a palliative care virtual simulation: A curricular short report. *Journal of Interprofessional Education & Practice*, *15*, 48–54.

Taubert, M., Webber, L., Hamilton, T., Carr, M., & Harvey, M. (2019). Virtual reality videos used in undergraduate palliative and oncology medical teaching: Results of a pilot study. *BMJ Supportive & Palliative Care*, *9*(3), 281–285.

10 Practical Skill Development

Introduction

With the exploration of various evidence-based VR interventions in previous chapters, the current chapter focuses on its clinical implementation. Aiming to address the multifaceted needs of patients, the VR interventions investigated in research vary significantly, and specific practical implementations must adhere to particular guidelines or protocols related to each VR intervention. This chapter offers clinical suggestions on the general use of VR interventions, such as retrieving VR videos from accessible online sources like *YouTube VR* app. Readers are encouraged to use these guidelines as a reference, tailoring their approach to the specific needs of each patient.

The chapter is divided into three sections, covering the essential steps before, during, and after VR interventions. The "Before VR Interventions" section elaborates on the equipment set-up, infection control, inviting patients for VR interventions, risk assessment, need assessment, and preparing the patient for VR interventions. The "During VR Interventions" section provides practical tips on patient engagement, interaction, and monitoring, while the "After VR Interventions" section outlines clinical strategies for a smooth transition and appropriate closure to VR sessions. The chapter aims to outline practical skills such that healthcare professionals can harness the potential of VR technology in their own clinical settings.

Before VR Interventions

Preparing a patient for any VR intervention is the essential and critical step for its quality delivery. This section elaborates on the preparation work prior to the delivery of VR interventions, which includes equipment set-up, infection control, inviting patients for VR interventions, risk assessment, need assessment, and preparing patients for VR interventions.

DOI: 10.4324/9781003518327-14

1.   *Equipment Set-up*

The basic VR equipment includes a VR headset and controller, VR camera, and cables for charging.

VR Headset and Controller

A standalone VR headset is used to increase portability in settings such as hospices and homes for older adults. The device is a head-mounted display with speakers to allow an immersive visual and auditory environment. The headset supports head tracking such that users would remain immersed with their head movements. The user interface uses that of common mobile devices (e.g., Android OS) on the market, operating with two hand-held motion sensing controllers.

VR Camera

A VR camera is a device designed to capture immersive 360-degree content for VR experiences. It allows users to record their own videos or images that can be viewed in VR headsets, smartphones, or computers, providing a more personalized viewing experience. It consists of multiple lenses to capture a 360-degree view. It allows capturing content in photo or video formats and live streams. Consumer-grade cameras available in the market and designed for capturing personal experiences or events are typically easy to use.

Internet Connection

The headset requires an internet connection for use with VR apps. To ensure a good internet connection, check the internet connection on "settings" and "network" in advance. If no stable network is available within the ward, the administrator may consider using a pocket Wi-Fi router.

VR Software

To maximize therapeutic potential while minimizing adverse effects associated with VR interventions, the following criteria are suggested for the selection of VR content or apps.

- VR content that caters to personal preferences and interests (see Chapter 1).
- Avoid VR content with elements that could potentially trigger anxiety, fear, or negative emotions in patients (Perna et al., 2021) unless special content, such as ghost houses and roller coasters, is requested.

- Avoid VR content with sudden head movements.
- Select VR content filmed with steady or stationary cameras to minimize sudden motions that can induce cybersickness.
- Select VR content with a lower intensity of visual disturbances, such as minimal use of rapid transitions.
- Select VR content that allows patients to focus on a fixed point or provides a stationary viewing experience.
- Avoid VR content that involves crowds, sudden unexpected noises, or sudden scene changes (Ferguson et al., 2020).

2. Infection Control

To ensure the safety and well-being of patients, it is essential to adhere to infection control measures. It is advised to maintain a sterile and hygienic environment to minimize the risk of cross contamination in clinical settings such as the spread of infectious diseases. The hygiene and infection control measures are suggested as follows.

- Prior to and after handling the VR headset and controllers, wash hands thoroughly with soap and water or use hand sanitizer to minimize the risk of cross-contamination.
- Between each use, sanitize the headset and controllers. Use non-abrasive anti-bacterial wipes to clean all components, and allow them to air dry completely before the next use. Ensure the wipe down along the hand controllers.
- Allow some time for the alcohol from the wipes to evaporate before using the headset again.
- If possible, use disposable or easily cleanable face masks or covers for VR headsets to reduce the risk of transmission of infectious diseases.
- Educate patients and palliative care providers on proper hand hygiene before and after VR sessions.

3. Inviting Patients for VR interventions

As VR may be a novel technology to most of the patients receiving palliative care, extending a respectful invitation to them is an essential step. It is foreseeable that patients' active participation and willingness to explore this innovative therapeutic approach can enhance the therapeutic impact of VR interventions. The invitation may include elements such as highlighting the evidence-based and patient-centred nature of VR interventions. In light of the clinical experiences of the author, this section provides a suggested invitation script and lists out the possible responses from patients with suggested approaches from therapists (Table 10.1).

Table 10.1 Possible responses from patients upon invitation and suggested responses

Possible Responses	Examples	Suggested Approach	Suggested Responses
Positive	"It sounds good. Let me try!"	• Acknowledge openness and willingness to try. • Prepare the patient for VR interventions (please refer to the section "Preparing Patient for VR Intervention").	"That's great to hear! VR can provide a new and engaging way to manage symptoms. I appreciate your eagerness to try something new."
Curiosity	"I've never heard of VR before. Can you tell me more about how it works?"	• Provide more details about VR interventions. • If possible, show the patient photos or videos of VR to help them understand more about VR before the VR experience.	"Of course! VR interventions involve using technology to create immersive experiences that can help to distract or relax your mind. It has shown promising results in symptom control such as pain and shortness of breath." "We can show you some photos of the VR headset and samples of VR content that may provide you with more ideas of what the VR technology is and how it operates for your consideration."
Apprehension	"I'm not sure if I'm comfortable with VR. It feels a bit overwhelming to me."	• Enquire about her concerns. Explore if the concern is physical or psychological in nature. • Address the concerns, e.g., weight problems, anxiety. • Reassure patient's concerns. • Provide room and space for the patient to make their decision with no pressure. Reassure that it's totally alright if he/she is not keen to try. • Respect the patient's decision.	"I understand that trying something new can be intimidating. We can locate VR content together that you mostly like, and we can start with gentle experiences. We can surely go at your own pace and ensure that you feel comfortable throughout the process." "What concerns you about using this new technology? Do you worry about any negative effects?"

(*Continued*)

Table 10.1 (Continued)

Possible Responses	Examples	Suggested Approach	Suggested Responses
Scepticism	*"I'm not convinced that VR interventions can alleviate my symptom distress. Are there any studies or evidence to support its effectiveness?"*	• Provide relevant studies with more concrete examples. • Reassure concerns. • Respect the patient's decision.	*"It's understandable to have questions. VR interventions have been studied extensively, and research suggests that virtual travel can help relieve pain and other symptoms. If preferred, I can provide you with the relevant publication paper."*
Fear	*"I'm afraid that VR interventions might worsen my symptoms or trigger anxiety."*	• Enquire further about potential concerns. • Address the concerns. • Reassure the patient that it's totally alright not to try VR interventions. • Respect the patient's decision.	*"I hear your concerns. Please be reassured that we always prioritize your comfort and safety. We can start with less intense experiences and gradually progress based on your feedback. Your well-being is our top priority, and we can adjust the interventions according to your needs. Please note that you will be in control during the whole virtual experience."* *"It is totally alright if you do not feel comfortable to try."*
Ambivalence/ Uninterested/ Unmotivated	*"I am too busy."* *"I am too tired."* *"I am not feeling particularly well today."*	• Explored underlying reasons. • Acknowledge concerns. • Respect the patient's decisions. • Provide alternatives.	*"Thank you for letting us know your concerns. Please take your time/take some rest."* *"If you do not mind, we might visit you another time to see if you are ready for VR intervention."*
Rejection	*"I don't think it helps; my condition remains the same after VR exposure."*	• Acknowledge the patient's sharing and concerns. • Respect the patient's decision.	*"Thank you for sharing your truthful thoughts. I understand that you have reservations. We can explore other approaches that may be deemed helpful to you."*

Suggested Invitation Script

Nice to meet you. I am [name] from the Department of [name]. Understanding that people here may experience a certain level of emotional or physical distress, we've brought along this virtual reality (VR) headset, which acts like a goggle that allows an immersive experience that virtually brings you to places you have fond memories of or doing things that you long to do, e.g., visiting your grandchildren in Canada, returning to a park that you used to go with your parents when small, or hiking. Scientific evidence shows that using this VR can help improve symptom control such as pain, mood, and anxiety and could also provide good opportunities for wish fulfilment. We wonder if there is any chance you would love to give it a try.

4. Risk Assessments

Pre-screening and risk assessment are essential components of the VR interventions to ensure patients' safety and well-being (Woo & Lee, 2023). It aims to minimize any potential harm to patients under the main principles of ethics—non-maleficence (Beauchamp & Childress, 2019)—highlighting the do-no-harm approach. This section begins with an overview of a list of suggested exclusion criteria, which serves as guides to screen out and exclude patients who may be at a higher risk of adverse effects of VR. It then proceeds with elaborating a range of assessment methods that enable healthcare professionals to collect comprehensive clinical information and to identify cognitively sound, mentally competent, emotionally stable, and physically fit patients who stand a higher chance to benefit from VR intervention.

Suggested Exclusion Criteria

- Significant visual and hearing impairment.
- Severe cognitive impairment.
- Patients with a history of epilepsy or having had a seizure in the past six weeks.
- Hypersensitivity to motion.
- Active nausea or vomiting.
- Physical disability such as neck injury.
- Current delirium symptoms.
- History of dissociative disorders.
- Currently in an active psychotic episode.
- Clinically depressed or unstable mood (Woo & Lee, 2023).
- Potential phobias or fears (Perna et al., 2021).
- Low degree of acceptance towards current illness condition (Woo & Lee, 2023).
- Low degree of psychological readiness to access virtual materials (Woo & Lee, 2023).

Assessment Methods

Effective assessment methods are essential for conducting thorough risk assessments prior to implementing tailored VR interventions for patients. This section introduces various assessment methods, including the review of medical records, patient interviews, and the collection of collateral information from caregivers and other healthcare professionals. The goal is to gain a comprehensive understanding of each patient's condition to minimize the potential risks of using VR interventions.

Reviewing Medical Record. In a clinical setting, medical records can be a helpful source for healthcare professionals to gather clinical information. Reviewing medical records can help identify any contraindications or precautions specific to individual patients. To assess the potential risks of individual patient in using VR interventions, the following items can be considered:

- Medical History. Medical history allows the identification of any pre-existing conditions that may impact their ability to engage in VR interventions safely. The pre-existing conditions include any diagnosis of epilepsy or having had a recent seizure, hypersensitivity to motion, active nausea or vomiting, and physical disability such as neck injury.
- Physical Health. The patient's physical health status, such as mobility, balance, and strength, might affect the patient's ability to use VR equipment. For instance, metastatic cancer with cord compression may limit one's sitting tolerance and use of a remote controller.
- Sensory Issues. Sensory impairments, such as visual or auditory deficits, may impact the patient's ability to fully experience and benefit from VR interventions. Obstacles and pitfalls may be encountered if sensory impairment is not known prior to VR interventions. Adjustment or accommodation may be needed to ensure full participation in the immersive experience of VR. For instance, patients may be advised to use their own glasses during VR interventions.
- Cognitive Functioning. VR interventions require a certain level of cognitive functioning to navigate and comprehend the virtual environment. It is essential to assess whether the patient has the capacity to understand and follow instructions during the VR experience. It is advised to understand the patient's cognitive abilities, such as alertness, orientation, attention, and short-term memory.
- Psychiatric diagnosis. There remains a chance that the immersive nature of VR interventions may aggravate clinical mood conditions, such as depression or anxiety. Woo and Lee (2023), in a perspective paper, highlight that VR exposure may pose psychological risks, including additional emotional distress if maladaptive cognitions of patients are triggered by

the virtual experience and not appropriately processed. For instance, underlying maladaptive cognitions related to regret or hopelessness may be triggered when recognizing that one might never be able to have such an experience in real life but only in a virtual context. It is, therefore, advised to assess in the medical record if there are any current or past psychiatric conditions or presentations of symptoms related to adjustment disorders, depressive disorders, anxiety disorders, trauma-related disorders, psychotic disorders, or dissociative disorders according to the diagnostic and statistical manual of mental disorders (DSM V, American Psychiatric Association, 2013).

Patient Interview. Individual interviews serve as a valuable opportunity to assess various aspects of a patient's mental and emotional state. In addition to verbal communication with patients, clinical information can be collected through behavioural observations of patients' non-verbal cues, such as eye contact, facial expressions, body language, and gestures. Healthcare professionals is advised to take note of any signs of discomfort, agitation, withdrawal, or other behavioural indicators that may suggest psychological or emotional distress prior to VR interventions. Healthcare professionals may directly ask patients the following aspects for risk assessments:

Delirium Symptoms. Delirium symptoms can be assessed on the patient's orientation to person, place, and time to take note of any confusion or disorientation prior to VR interventions (Table 10.2).

Clinically Depressed or Unstable Mood. The interview aims to collect additional or supplementary information to that obtained from patients' medical record. It allows for an assessment of present mental and mood conditions based on the symptoms outlined in the DSM-V (American Psychiatric Association, 2013). As VR offers an immersive experience that creates a strong sense of presence (McCreery et al., 2013), VR exposure

Table 10.2 Suggested interview questions on delirium symptoms

Orientations	Suggested interview questions
Person	Can you please tell me your full name? Do you know who I am?
Place	Do you know where you are right now? Do you know which city/town you are in? What is the name of this building?
Time	What is the current year? Can you tell me the current season or month? What is the date/week of today?

can potentially activate underlying maladaptive cognitions in some patients. If these cognitions are not effectively processed or addressed, they can lead to further emotional turbulence (Woo & Lee, 2023). This evaluation helps identify patients who may require timely psychological support or intervention before engaging in VR interventions.

Psychotic Episode. VR demands patients who are in good contact with reality. VR interventions are thus not recommended for patients with acute psychosis in a palliative care setting. Healthcare professionals should provide an assessment of the presence of hallucinations or delusions so as to determine if patients have good reality-testing abilities. If active psychotic symptoms are present, patients would benefit from immediate psychiatric intervention more than VR for the time being. Despite the limited empirical evidence, patients with a history of psychotic symptoms who are currently in remission and presenting with a stable mood may be eligible for VR experiences, provided there are no other contraindications.

Degree of Acceptance towards Current Condition. Healthcare professionals can assess the patient's degree of acceptance towards their current palliative condition (Table 10.3). It helps gauge the patient's psychological readiness to engage with VR interventions, during which the patient may virtually travel to a dream place one longs to visit with a healthy identity. Individuals with low acceptance towards palliative status, such as patients still hoping for curative treatment despite their palliative condition, may not be able to endure the emotional distress or disappointment that arises (Woo & Lee, 2023).

Psychological Readiness for VR Interventions. The lack of readiness for VR experiences may pose additional psychological risks (Woo & Lee, 2023). To minimize potential harm, healthcare professionals can evaluate the patient's psychological readiness to engage with virtual materials during the interview. It can be assessed on one's willingness to explore new technologies, openness to try new approaches, any previous experiences with VR, expectations towards VR interventions, and other related concerns (Table 10.4).

Table 10.3 Suggested interview questions on the degree of acceptance

	Suggested interview questions
Emotional Response	*How do you feel about the current incurable status? Do you feel angry, sad, or frustrated?* *How have you been coping with the current condition so far?*
VR expectations	*Do you anticipate any emotional distress in the transition from the ideal virtual world back to the real-world situation after VR interventions?*

Table 10.4 Suggested interview questions on psychological readiness for VR interventions

	Suggested Interview Questions
Motivation and Willingness	Are you willing to try VR as a potential tool for managing your symptoms? The virtual experience that you have chosen may trigger your past memories. Are you ready for that?
Openness to New Approaches	How comfortable are you with using new technology, such as smartphones, computers, or VR devices?
Familiarity with Technology	Have you had any previous/negative experiences with VR or similar technologies?
Expectations	What specific outcomes or benefits are you hoping to achieve through VR interventions?
Comfort Level	Are there any concerns or reservations you have about using VR?

Table 10.5 Suggested interview questions when collecting collateral information

	Suggested Interview Questions
Concerns	Do you have any concerns if this patient tries novel VR interventions for symptom management? Do you anticipate any problems or difficulties if this patient engages in such a novel technology?
Personal Opinions	In light of your expertise and understanding of this patient, do you advise her/him to try the VR interventions?

Collateral information. It is helpful to collect collateral information from various sources, such as caregivers and healthcare professionals in the clinical settings, including physicians, physiotherapists, occupational therapists, social workers, and chaplains. Their prior communication with and understanding towards patients may provide information about the patient's pre-existing conditions that may impact their suitability for VR interventions (Table 10.5).

5. Need Assessments

Need assessment is deemed essential, though often omitted, prior to VR interventions. It is based on the premise that VR intervention may bring harm to those who do not need it. It involves evaluating and prioritizing the specific needs, preferences, and goals of an individual patient. Conducting need assessments may provide the added benefit of identifying alternative interventions or approaches that may be more suitable for patients who do not require or may even be at risk from VR interventions. For instance, the patient may only need more factual information on advance care planning rather than symptom management through VR interventions at a certain time point. The need assessment then ensures that resources and interventions are allocated appropriately to minimize potential adverse effects. It aligns with the ethical principle of do-no-harm and patient-centred approach that allows healthcare professionals to develop personalized care plans to address the unique needs and preferences of an individual patient.

Assessment Methods

Similar to risk assessments, clinical information related to a patient's needs can be collected through various sources, including medical records, patient interviews, and standardized assessments.

Reviewing Medical Record. To assess a patient's individual needs through medical records, the following items can be considered:

- Physical needs: Examine the documentation of any specific symptoms experienced by the patient, such as pain, shortness of breath, and fatigue.
- Psychological needs: Examine the documentation of any specific mood symptoms such as anxiety, depression, and coping strategies.
- Social needs: Examine the documentation of any needs for support from family and friends.
- Spiritual needs: Examine the documentation of any spiritual beliefs or religions.

Intake Interview. The intake interview serves as a valuable platform to directly ask patients about their most imminent needs that VR intervention can cater to (Table 10.6). It is ideal to create a safe and supportive environment where

Table 10.6 Suggested interview questions on need assessments

	Suggested Interview Questions
Physical Needs	Are you experiencing any physical discomfort, such as pain and fatigue?
Psychological Needs	Do you feel anxious, negative/gloomy, or bored? Are there any places that you have always dreamt of visiting but have not the opportunity? Are there any places that you would like to revisit?
Social Needs	Are there any family members or friends whom you would like to express your feelings or thoughts to? Are there any social events that you would like to participate in?
Spiritual Needs	Are there any religious rituals or practices that you would like to engage in? Do you want to participate virtually in some church events? Do you have any past memories you want to revisit?
Personal Priorities	Which specific symptoms/needs that you would like to prioritize or focus on at this juncture?

patients feel comfortable directly expressing their needs, concerns, desires, and priorities. Such an approach aligns with the patient-centred principle that respects individual differences and autonomy.

Standardized Assessment Tools. Standardized assessment tools provide a systematic and evidence-based approach to gathering information about the patient's needs. It helps monitor patients' symptom changes before and after VR interventions. It also helps assess the effectiveness of VR interventions in symptom management and make informed decisions about the appropriateness and potential benefits of VR for individual patients. Examples of some standardized assessment tools are suggested in Table 10.7.

6. Preparing Patient for VR Intervention

Prior to VR interventions, preparing patients for VR intervention is an essential step, as patients may be new to such technology. This subsection suggests clinical guidelines to ensure patients are well-informed and ready to

Table 10.7 Suggested assessment tools

	Suggested Assessment Tools
Physical and Psychological Needs	**Edmonton Symptom Assessment System (ESAS)** (Bruera et al., 1991). ESAS is a commonly used outcome measure that measures the severity of nine symptoms commonly experienced by patients with cancer. The nine symptoms are pain, tiredness, nausea, depression, anxiety, drowsiness, appetite, well-being, and shortness of breath. Each item is rated on a numerical scale from 0 to 10, with 10 indicating *Most severe.* If a patient, for example, reports high levels of pain, anxiety, or fatigue, VR interventions targeting relaxation, distraction, or pain management may be considered.
Social Needs	**The UCLA Loneliness Short Scale** (Hughes et al., 2004) is an abbreviated version of the 20-item Revised UCLA Loneliness Scale (Russell et al., 1980). This 3-item scale is used to assess the extent of loneliness experienced by individuals, specifically by asking how frequently they perceive a lack of companionship, feel excluded, and sense isolation from others. For VR content that may facilitate a sense of "social presence" or communication with family members, this scale may help assess the change in the sense of loneliness.
Spiritual Needs	**The Functional Assessment of Chronic Illness Therapy** (Webster et al., 1999) is a collection of health-related quality-of-life questionnaires targeted to the management of chronic illness. The spiritual well-being subscale (Peterman et al., 2002) from this inventory is a validated questionnaire designed to measure various aspects of spirituality and faith that contribute to improving the quality of life for individuals with chronic illnesses. The scale consists of 12 items that are categorized into three domains: meaning, peace, and faith (Canada et al., 2008; Murphy et al., 2010; Peterman et al., 2014). Each item is rated on a numerical scale from 0 to 4, with 0 indicating *Not at all* and 4 indicating *Very much.*

engage in VR sessions safely and comfortably. The guideline aims to create a supportive environment that maximizes the therapeutic benefits while minimizing any potential risks associated with VR interventions. What follows is suggested verbal script.

- Ensure that the patient is at a comfortable posture prior to and during VR interventions, which may last for 5–10 minutes.
- Educate patients about possible side effects and symptoms (e.g., cybersickness, possible emotional distress when transitioning from VR) during and after VR sessions.
- Reassure patients that the offer of breaks during VR sessions to minimize any physical or emotional discomfort.
- Reassure our empathetic presence and company during the whole VR experience.
- Establish a gesture or verbal signal with patients such that they can indicate termination in case of any discomfort.
- Facilitate a sense of control throughout the VR experience by reassuring patients that the virtual experience can be terminated anytime.
- Encourage patients to share feedback on the VR experiences during or after VR sessions.
- Reassure the patient that some grounding work, if needed, can be carried out after VR interventions to ensure a smooth transition from virtuality to reality.
- Brief patients that they can move their heads for the immersive experience during the VR intervention.

Suggested Script

Before our VR journey, please kindly let me share more information to prepare you well for the VR experience. Some users may experience motion sickness, eye strain, or other discomfort. To minimize the risk, we have limited the VR experience to 10 minutes and chosen VR content that is of higher quality. If there is any chance you notice any physical or emotional discomfort, please let us know immediately. Please make sure the current posture is comfortable to you.

Throughout the VR experience, it's important to listen to your body and pace yourself. If you feel the need to pause, please let us know directly. We may now establish a gesture or signal (for example, waving hands or saying "stop") to indicate session termination. This ensures that you always have control over your experience and can communicate your needs even while immersed in the virtual environment. I will be here throughout the VR experience. It would be great if you could share with me your thoughts or feelings during the VR experience.

Moreover, you can move your head to see your left or right side to feel more immersed in the virtual environment. Most VR users do not experience discomfort but the awe and joy of virtual travel to a desired place. Do you have any questions? Please relax and enjoy.

During VR Intervention

During VR interventions, mental health professionals play a vital role in enhancing the therapeutic experience and ensuring patient comfort. This section provides several clinical tips that therapists can employ. These tips target patient engagement, interaction, and monitoring. Table 10.8 lists the possible responses from patients during VR and suggested approaches for handling such responses.

1. Patient Engagement

- Encourage the patient to immerse themselves in the virtual environment by guiding questions such as, *"Please relax and look around you," "Please feel free to explore the environment."*
- Assist the patient in holding the VR headset to decrease subjective weight.
- Prompt the patient to describe the virtual scenario in detail, further engaging them with the content and here-and-now. Prompting questions such as, *"What is in front of you?," " What are you seeing now?," "How are you feeling?," or "What is the colour of the sky?"*
- Allow the patient to freely express their feelings or thoughts.

2. VR Experience and Interaction

- Encourage patients to move their heads to explore the 180-degree view, facilitating their sense of control and presence.
- Respond to the patient's expression of feelings or thoughts with simple acknowledgment or reflection. May consider simply repeating their expressions or statements to show empathy and provide a sense of companionship. Please refer to Table 10.8 for the possible responses in patients and suggested responses during their VR interventions.
- Actively listen to the patient's ideas, thoughts, and sharing, which can help identify personal interests and values and facilitate further interaction during or after VR interventions. Encourage further sharing after VR interventions if the condition allows.

Table 10.8 Possible responses from patients during VR

Possible Responses	Examples	Suggested Approach	Suggested Responses
Enjoyment	*"Wow! I see the fishes here in the deep sea! They look so cute . . . the turtles too . . . . Oh, what is this creature? It is so amazing!"*	• Allow time for description and expression of feelings. • Facilitate more description for the here-and-now moment. • Reflect emotions, if appropriate. • Repeat the patient's expression to reassure them of the therapist's presence in the venture.	• *"Yes, the fishes look cute. So do the turtles."* • *"They are so amazing."* • *"We are curious about the sea world."* • *"What colour are they?"* • *"What are your feelings now?"* • *"What is the colour of the fish?"*
Relief	*"It is such a calming place!"* *"Wow, I like this!"*	• Allow time for description and expression of feelings. • Reflect emotions, if appropriate. • Repeat the patient's expression to reassure them of the therapist's presence in the venture.	• *"It is a peaceful place."* • *"It brings us a sense of calmness."* • *"We like being in such a calming place."* • *"Any thoughts coming up to your mind now?"* • *"Please tell me more about what you are seeing."*
Discomfort	*"Ugh, I am a bit queasy and dizzy."*	• Terminate the VR intervention immediately. • Reassure that the patient's comfort is the top priority. • Provide options for symptom control, e.g., offering relaxation coaching, allowing time for rest.	*"I am sorry to hear that VR is making you feel queasy and dizzy. That's definitely not the goal. Let's take a break and discuss some adjustments we can make to help you feel better."* *"We can continue or discontinue, dependent on your preferences."*
Overwhelm	*"The VR environment is too intense for me. It's triggering my anxiety."*	• Terminate the VR intervention immediately. • Reassure that the patient's readiness and preference is the priority. • Provide options for anxiety management, e.g., relaxation.	*"I totally understand. VR can be pretty intense and overwhelming. We want to make sure it's a helpful tool, not a source of distress. We can discontinue the VR interventions. If you prefer, we can perform some relaxation to help lower the anxiety."*
Boredom	*"I'm finding the VR experience too dull, boring, and unengaging. It's not helping me with symptom control."*	• Terminate the VR intervention immediately. • Acknowledge the patient's genuine sharing and openness to trying new treatment approaches. • Reassure and validate emotions. • Explore if other virtual environments may be preferred. • Respect the patient's choice. • Reassure them of the availability of alternative approaches for symptom control/to meet their needs.	*"Thanks for sharing your honest feedback about finding VR boring. It's important to have activities that resonate with you. We can end today's VR session right away. It is also alright if you remain keen to explore other VR content that could be more engaging and meaningful to you."*

A Case Sharing

- A patient expresses his wish to virtually travel in an underwater world. He began to spontaneously express his own feelings and thoughts during the deep sea diving experience: "water flow is speedy," "this fish is rare!," "I like studying the underwater world," suggesting his familiarity and connection with the sea. He continues to share that "because I grew up in the sea," which further reinforces that the patient's life has been closely tied to the marine environment. During VR interventions, clinical techniques such as reflections or rephrasing his expressions may facilitate his continual expressions while at the same time reassuring them of the therapist's presence in his VR venture.
- These expressions facilitate a richer understanding of his life experience. After the VR exposure, such understanding provides a good starting point to continue meaningful discussion on his past life experiences, his sea-related wisdom, and his interest in the underwater, all of which may facilitate life review interventions building on his own life narrative and strengths.

3. *Monitoring and Adjusting VR Interventions*

- Monitor patients for signs of fatigue or discomfort and adjust session durations accordingly.
- Continually evaluate the effectiveness and safety of VR interventions based on patients' feedback and facilitators' ongoing assessment during the VR session.
- Be attentive to any indications of physical risks and adjust interventions accordingly.
- Be prepared to terminate the VR interventions when the patient shows signs of physical or emotional discomfort.

After VR Interventions

The literature has documented psychological difficulties in readjusting to the real world after VR interventions, often accompanied by a sense of the real world feeling unreal (Behr et al., 2005; Woo & Lee, 2023). It is, therefore, essential to ensure a smooth transition for patients from the virtual world back to reality. This phase requires careful guidance and support to help patients ground themselves and adjust well to their physical surroundings. This section outlines the clinical tips that aim to facilitate the patient's smooth transition and provide appropriate closure to VR sessions as a whole. Table 10.9 lists possible responses from patients after VR and the suggested responsive approach from the VR facilitators.

Table 10.9 Possible responses from patients after VR

Possible Responses	Examples	Suggested Approach	Suggested Responses
Positive Response	"That VR experience was incredible! I feel so much better and more relaxed. I really like it!"	• Acknowledge strength, e.g., willingness to try new treatment approaches, quick learning of new technology, and receptive to technological support. • Deliver psychoeducation, e.g., positive activities facilitate physical and emotional symptom control. • If possible, allow further discussions based on the VR experiences to explore personal values or meanings, paving the way for life review interventions or acceptance and commitment therapy. • Invite patients for more VR sessions.	• "I'm most joyful to hear that the VR experience had such a positive impact on you! It's great to see how it helps to improve your symptom control. I appreciate your strength in trying a new treatment approach and advanced technology." • "In light of your VR experience, we learn that what we do affects how we feel physically and emotionally. We can indeed play an active role in managing our symptoms." • "If you are keen, we can prepare for more VR sessions."
Mixed Response	"I had mixed feelings about the VR session. It was interesting, but I feel a bit tired now."	• Reassure patient's concerns. • Allow resting time. • Follow-up session to assess their tiredness after VR and to make adjustments if the patient prefers more VR sessions.	• "Thank you for sharing your thoughts. It's understandable to have mixed feelings. Let's take some rest first and discuss more a bit now or later as you prefer." • "Let's dive deeper into your VR experience to better understand what aspects worked for you and what didn't. Given that you find the VR experience interesting, how about we have shorter VR duration for the next time if you are keen for more VR sessions?"
Neutral or Negative Response	"Honestly, I didn't really notice any change in my symptoms after the VR session. It was a bit underwhelming." "VR just isn't for me. I didn't enjoy the experience, and it didn't do anything for my symptoms."	• Acknowledge the patient's feedback. • Reassure concerns. • Appreciate patient's willingness to try. • If possible, explore possible factors underlying the lack of positive outcome, e.g., appropriateness of the virtual content, quality of VR video, unmatched expectations.	• "I appreciate your honesty and understand that VR might not be the right fit for everyone. Let's explore other treatment options that align more with your preferences and goals. We can find alternative approaches that have proven effectiveness in symptom control."

1. **Smooth Transition from Virtual to Real World**

- Prepare patient for the closure near the end of VR experience.

  - *"We've just been immersed in a VR experience that may have felt very real. We are about to end our virtual experiences and are now preparing you to return to reality. I will remove the headset a while later [pause]."*
  - *"Please close your eyes and take a deep breath [pause]."*

- If needed, use grounding techniques to help patients reorient themselves near the end of the VR experience or after the removal of the VR headset.

  - *"As you close your eyes, let's take a moment to ground ourselves [pause]."*
  - *"Take a deep breath in through your nose and exhale gently through your mouth [pause]. Attend to your breath. Feel the natural rhythm of your breath. Breathe in and out [pause] in and out [pause] in and out [long pause] . . . ."*
  - *"Bring your attention to your lower body. Feel the weight of your body on the chair/bed. Notice the support beneath you [pause]."*
  - *"Turn your focus to the sounds around you. Notice the gentle hum of the environment, such as the white noise from the air-conditioner in the room [pause]."*
  - *"Begin to move your fingers. Feel the sensation of movement in your fingers."*
  - *"Slowly open your eyes and take a moment to adjust to the light [pause]."*
  - *"Look at the room [pause], the wall [pause], and the ceiling [pause]."*

- Verbally orient the patient after removal of the headset.

  - *"Right now, you are in [location]. You are sitting in a comfortable chair (or lying in bed)."*
  - *"Take a moment to relax and allow your mind to come back to the reality [pause]."*

- Observe the patient's facial expression and body. Ask a few questions to ensure a smooth transition.

  - *"How are you feeling right now?"*
  - *"Are you experiencing any discomfort or uneasiness?"*
  - *"Did you notice any difficulties in shifting your awareness from the virtual environment to the physical surroundings?"*
  - *"Are there any lingering effects or sensations from the VR experience that you would like to discuss or share?"*

- Inquire if the patient would like to try the VR experience again and explore their reasons for wanting or not wanting to do so.

  - *"Are you interested in trying VR again?"*
  - *"Are there any specific reasons why you might be hesitant or reserved about trying the VR experience again?"*

- *"Do you feel that the VR experience provided any positive outcomes for you? If so, could you share what those were?"*

- Prepare to provide timely psychological interventions if the patient experiences any emotional distress or presents any maladaptive cognitions after the virtual experiences.
- In case of any signs of dissociative or disoriented symptoms, such as confusion, detachment from their surroundings, or difficulty grounding themselves, after VR interventions:

  - First of all, maintain a calm and reassuring demeanor.
  - Try to provide a comforting and safe environment for the patient to minimize further external stimuli for a sense of safety and familiarity.
  - Prepare to employ grounding techniques, guiding the patient to engage their senses and focus on the present moment.
  - Encourage the patient to verbalize their experiences, emotions, and any lingering feelings of disorientation or dissociation.
  - Seek professional help if necessary, such as a referral to a clinical psychologist or psychiatrist to ensure appropriate clinical support and treatment.

2. *Termination of VR Session*

To facilitate successful termination, a VR session should end with mutual agreement. A few clinical tips are provided in what follows.

- Assess the patient's readiness for ending the VR session by considering their subjective reports of satisfaction and overall comfort. Please refer to Table 10.9 for the possible responses from patients after VR interventions. Suggested assessment questions include:

  - *"How would you rate your level of satisfaction with the VR experience, with 1 indicating least satisfied while 10 being highly satisfied?"*
  - *"On a scale of 0–10, how would you rate your level of comfort during the VR experience?"*
  - *"From 0 to 10, to what extent do you feel like your physical, psychological, social, or spiritual needs are met through this VR experience?"*
  - *"Do you agree that the outcomes are what you were hoping for?"*

- Review the progress and discuss any insights, challenges, or achievements that may emerge.

  - *"Did you find the VR session enjoyable? Were there any specific moments or aspects that stood out to you?"*

- *"Were there any parts of the VR experience that you found challenging or uncomfortable?"*
- *"Is there anything you would like to explore or address further before concluding the VR session?"*

- Understand that some patients may experience a sense of attachment to the virtual environment or difficulties transitioning back to reality. Address their concerns and explore their thoughts and feelings about concluding the VR session.
- Provide time for reflection within the VR session, allowing the patient to process their experiences and emotions related to the virtual environment.
- Consider more VR sections upon the patient's request
- If possible, schedule a follow-up session for the patient a few days or a week after to evaluate any comments or effects.

3. Therapists' Reflection on Termination

- Emphasize the progress made by the patient during the VR session, highlighting their strengths, achievements, and growth.
- Take the opportunity to deliver psychoeducation on the inter-relationships among our behavior, thoughts, emotions, and bodily responses. Encourage similar positive activities during the illness journey.
- Encourage the patient to carry forward the lessons and experiences from the VR session into their everyday life. For example, if VR interventions on relaxation are well received, patients can be encouraged to practise traditional relaxation or view related videos, e.g., YouTube relaxation videos.

Table 10.10 Suggested self-reflective questions for VR facilitators

Theme	Reflection Questions
Prioritizing Patient Needs	• Did I make sure the virtual experience was truly centred on enhancing the patient's quality of life rather than any other agenda or motivation, such as an institute's preference of using new technology like VR and the personal motivation of "doing good" to patients? • Have I put forth an effort to actively elicit and consider the patient's feedback throughout the VR intervention? • Did I consider the patient's values, needs, preferences, interests, cultural background, and spiritual beliefs when selecting VR content?
Balancing Needs and Outcomes	• Are there any instances where my own needs or goals (e.g., to do good, to achieve a successful outcome) took precedence over the patient's expressed needs and preferences?

(*Continued*)

Table 10.10 (Continued)

Theme	Reflection Questions
	• How would I navigate situations where the patient's needs conflicted with my own professional objectives for delivering VR interventions? For instance, when a doctor specializing in palliative care prefers VR interventions for patients who show limited or no interest. • Have I ever felt the need to "push" the patient to engage with the VR therapy, thinking that VR interventions would be therapeutic to patients?
Underlying Fears and Concerns	• Do I have any underlying fears or hesitations about inviting the patient to try the VR interventions, such as a fear of rejection or uncertainty about their response? If so, how did I address or overcome these concerns? • What strategies do I have to build trust and comfort with the patient so that they feel ready and willing to engage with the VR technology? • Do I have any preconceived notions or biases about the patient's willingness or ability to use VR technology, such as younger patients more likely willing to play with VR and patients in general are happy to try exciting and novel technology? • How do I make sure the patient has realistic expectations towards VR intervention?
Promoting Beneficence and Non-Maleficence	• Have I put forth my best effort to minimize unintended harm or adverse effects? • Am I mindful of any contraindications or potential risk factors that may bring harm to the patient during VR interventions? • Am I aware that VR intervention, in certain extent, needs collaboration and communication with the palliative care team to ensure the VR therapy aligned with the overall palliative care plan? • Am I familiar with the contingency plan in case of adverse effects arising from VR interventions? • Am I ready to share with patients the possible negative reactions or adverse effects that could arise from VR therapy?
Ethical Considerations	• Do I have an ethical mindset when delivering VR interventions to patients who are most vulnerable in their end-of-life journey? • Am I aware of the various ethical principles, such as autonomy, beneficence, non-maleficence, and justice in the delivery of the VR interventions? • Am I alert of the patient's privacy and confidentiality, which should always be protected throughout the VR intervention?

- If comfortable, reflect on your own thoughts and feelings as a VR facilitator during the termination phase of the session. Please refer to Table 10.10 for the personal reflection questions. VR facilitators may consider providing feedback to patients, such as sharing their own feelings or appreciation for the patient's personal strengths, like openness to try new interventions.

Conclusions

This chapter covers the suggested steps before, during, and after VR interventions, outlining practical skills aimed at maximizing the benefits while minimizing the potential adverse effects of applying VR in patients during their end-of-life stage. Furthermore, this chapter aspires to serve as a solid starting point for healthcare professionals who may have limited knowledge about VR implementation in palliative care. It provides concrete and actionable suggestions, hoping to enhance understanding and increase confidence in using VR technology effectively and ethically to improve palliative care.

References

American Psychiatric Association. (2013). *Diagnostic and statistical manual of mental disorders: DSM-5* (5th ed.). American Psychiatric Association. https://doi.org/10.1176/appi.books.9780890425596

Beauchamp, T. L., & Childress, J. F. (2019). *Principles of biomedical ethics* (8th ed.). Oxford University Press.

Behr, K.-M., Nosper, A., Klimmt, C., & Hartmann, T. (2005). Some practical considerations of ethical issues in VR research. *Presence, 14*, 668–676.

Bruera, E., Kuehn, N., Miller, M., Selmser, P., & Macmillan, K. (1991). The Edmonton symptom assessment system (ESAS): A simple method for the assessment of palliative care patients. *Journal of Palliative Care, 7*, 6–9. https://doi.org/10.1177/082585979100700202

Canada, A. L., Murphy, P. E., Fitchett, G., Peterman, A. H., & Schover, L. R. (2008). A 3-factor model for the FACIT-Sp. *Psycho-Oncology, 17*(9), 908–916.

Ferguson, C., Shade, M. Y., Blaskewicz Boron, J., Lyden, E., & Manley, N. A. (2020). Virtual reality for therapeutic recreation in dementia hospice care: A feasibility study. *American Journal of Hospice & Palliative Medicine, 37*(10), 809–815. https://doi.org/10.1177/1049909120901525

Hughes, M. E., Waite, L. J., Hawkley, L. C., & Cacioppo, J. T. (2004). A short scale for measuring loneliness in large surveys: Results from two population-based studies. *Research on Aging, 26*(6), 655–672. https://doi.org/10.1177/0164027504268574

McCreery, M., Schrader, P., Krach, S., & Boone, R. (2013). A sense of self: The role of presence in virtual environments. *Computers in Human Behavior, 29*(4), 1635–1640.

Murphy, P. E., Canada, A. L., Fitchett, G., Stein, K., Portier, K., Crammer, C., & Peterman, A. H. (2010). An examination of the 3-factor model and structural invariance across racial/ethnic groups for the FACIT-Sp: A report from the American cancer society's study of cancer survivors-II (SCS-II). *Psycho-Oncology, 19*(3), 264–272.

Perna, L., Lund, S., White, N., & Minton, O. (2021). The potential of personalized virtual reality in palliative care: A feasibility trial. *American Journal of Hospice & Palliative Medicine, 38*(12), 1488–1494. https://doi.org/10.1177/1049909121994299

Peterman, A. H., Fitchett, G., Brady, M. J., Hernandez, L., & Cella, D. (2002). Measuring spiritual wellbeing in people with cancer: The functional assessment of chronic illness therapy? Spiritual wellbeing scale (FACIT-Sp). *Annals of Behavioral Medicine, 24*(1), 49–58.

Peterman, A. H., Reeve, C. L., Winford, E. C., Cotton, S., Salsman, J. M., McQuellon, R., Tsevat, J., & Campbell, C. (2014). Measuring meaning and peace with the FACIT–spiritual well-being scale: Distinction without a difference? *Psychological Assessment, 26*(1), 127–137.

Russell, D., Peplau, L., & Cutrona, C. (1980). The revised UCLA loneliness scale: Concurrent and discriminant validity evidence. *Journal of Personality and Social Psychology, 39*(3), 472–480.

Webster, K., Odom, L., Peterman, A., Lent, L., & Cella, D. (1999). The functional assessment of chronic illness therapy (FACIT) measurement system: Validation of version 4 of the core questionnaire. *Quality of Life Research, 8*(7), 604.

Woo, O. K. L., & Lee, A. M. (2023). A perspective on potential psychological risks and solutions of using virtual reality in palliative care. *Frontiers in Virtual Reality, 4.* https://doi.org/10.3389/frvir.2023.1256641

Section IV

Ethical Considerations

This section focuses on the ethical considerations surrounding the use of VR in clinical practice. It explores the challenges and potential risks associated with VR interventions and the importance of professional training for its clinical use. Chapter 11 introduces the physical and psychological risks that may arise when VR interventions do not work out as intended, highlighting the importance of monitoring and addressing any adverse effects on patients' well-being. Chapter 12 discusses the professional training required for the clinical use of VR, emphasizing the need for specialized knowledge, skills, and attitudes in this clinical field.

DOI: 10.4324/9781003518327-15

11 Physical and Psychological Risks of Virtual Reality Interventions

Introduction

The concept of technology as "Faustian bargains," coined by Postman (1995), suggests that certain moral, ethical, or spiritual values are often compromised in exchange for wealth, power, or other advantages. This notion may hold true when considering the use of VR among patients facing existential crises. In the realm of biomedical ethics (Beauchamp & Childress, 2019), the principle of *beneficence* emphasizes the importance of pursuing positive therapeutic outcomes that serve the best interests of patients. Considering the compelling evidence supporting the use of VR interventions in patients receiving palliative care in previous chapters, VR appears to be a beneficial intervention that warrants widespread utilization. While there is recognition of VR's potential benefits, it is important to acknowledge that along with the numerous benefits, the application of VR in palliative care also presents certain risks, both physical and psychological, that need to be carefully considered and addressed. With the possibilities of potential risks and therefore moral concerns that without special precautions may harm patients, the delivery of VR intervention may violate another ethical principle of *non-maleficence* (Beauchamp & Childress, 2019).

This chapter accordingly shifts a focus towards exploring the risks associated with VR interventions, aiming to provide a comprehensive understanding of these risks and offer practical recommendations to mitigate them. The first half of the chapter focuses on discussing the physical risks, including motion sickness, eye strain, tripping/falls, sensory overload, pre-existing medical conditions, infection, and pre-existing injuries. Each risk will be examined in detail, followed by a set of recommendations to mitigate these risks. The second half of the chapter discusses the psychological risk factors for emotional distress in the use of VR interventions, including underlying maladaptive cognitions, clinical mood problems, low degree of acceptance towards current status, low degree of readiness for VR content, and reentry

DOI: 10.4324/9781003518327-16

problems. Similarly, recommendations will be provided to reduce the potential psychological risks.

Physical Risks and Recommendations

VR technology, although immersive and engaging, can lead to various physical challenges and discomfort for patients. This section focuses on exploring the physical risks associated with VR interventions in palliative care.

Motion Sickness

Motion sickness, often referred to as cybersickness in the context of VR, is a common side effect of VR, especially when there is a disconnect between the visual stimuli provided by the VR headset and the user's physical movement (Baniasadi et al., 2020). Some individuals may experience symptoms such as dizziness, nausea, and disorientation, which can be distressing for patients already dealing with physical discomfort (Weech et al., 2019). These symptoms are often triggered by errors in position tracking, optical distortion, flicker, inadequate resolution, delays in transport, or low update rates (Kennedy et al., 2000).

Eye Strain and Fatigue

Prolonged use of VR headsets can cause eye strain and fatigue (Smith & Burd, 2019). The close proximity of the display to the eyes and the prolonged exposure to virtual images can lead to eye discomfort, dryness, and fatigue (Sheppard & Wolffsohn, 2018). Szpak et al. (2019) report that after 30 minutes of use of head-mounted displays, some individuals experience symptoms of blurred vision, diplopia, and sore eyes. Other studies find that VR headsets lead to higher visual fatigue compared to the use of PCs, tablets, or smartphones (Han et al., 2017; Souchet et al., 2018; Yu et al., 2018; Zhang et al., 2020).

Tripping and Falls

When using VR, individuals may become less aware of their physical surroundings. This can increase the risk of tripping, falling, or colliding with objects in the real environment (Levy et al., 2016). The motion sickness and postural instability induced by VR use might increase the risk of falls among older adults (Horlings et al., 2008; Riccio & Stoffregen, 1991; Weech et al., 2019). In a palliative care setting where patients may already be frail or have limited mobility, this risk should be carefully considered.

Sensory Overload

VR can create a highly immersive and stimulating experience by engaging multiple senses. Such visual and audio displays may result in information overload. *Information overload* refers to "the moment when the amount of available information exceeds the user's ability to process it" (Klapp, 1982, p. 63). It is found to be associated with stress levels, health issues, emotional distress, disillusionment, depression, and suboptimal decision-making (Edmunds & Morris, 2000; Helmersen et al., 2001). It may be particularly overwhelming for those who are sensitive to bright lights, loud sounds, or intense visual stimuli. People with autism spectrum disorder might be hypersensitive to sensory inputs, in which the use of VR might be aversive and distressing (Schmidt et al., 2021; Thye et al., 2018).

Pre-existing Medical Conditions

Patients with certain pre-existing medical conditions, such as epilepsy or cardiac issues, may be more susceptible to adverse effects when using VR. The flashing lights and rapid movements in VR content can potentially trigger seizures or exacerbate cardiovascular symptoms. A review study has warned about the risk of inducing photosensitive seizures among patients with epilepsy when the VR content contains bright flashes, provocative patterns, or colour changes (Fisher et al., 2022).

Pre-existing Injury

The use of VR might cause muscle fatigue and discomfort in supporting the weight of the device, potentially causing tension around the neck and shoulder areas (Kim & Shin, 2018; Penumudi et al., 2020; Yan et al., 2019). Some individuals may experience back pain when using head-mounted display devices (Botella et al., 2016). Prolonged and repeated use of VR might also carry a risk for repetitive strain injury (van Tulder et al., 2007). Careful consideration of patients' pre-existing injuries, such as wounds on the upper body and back pain, is needed to prevent the exacerbation of these conditions.

Infection

The use of medical devices in a healthcare setting could lead to nosocomial transmission and outbreaks if they are used without proper disinfection and sterilization procedures (Rutala & Weber, 2016). The use of VR devices in healthcare settings might unintentionally transmit pathogens between patients and staff, creating a risk of spreading infectious diseases.

VR equipment particularly warrants concerns given its proximity to user's mucus membranes, including nose, mouth, and eyes, and its reusable nature among multiple users (Moore et al., 2021). In particular, certain VR equipment contains porous surfaces, which are more difficult to disinfect compared to nonporous surfaces, leading to an elevated risk of transmitting diseases (Roberts et al., 2022).

Recommendations

- **Perform a thorough pre-screening and risk assessment of patients** to identify any pre-existing conditions or physical limitations that may increase the risk of adverse effects from VR (Behr et al., 2005).
- **Establish clear exclusion criteria** to identify patients who may be at higher risk for experiencing adverse physical effects from VR (Chapter 10). Consider factors such as history of epilepsy, physical injuries, or hypersensitivity to motions when determining the suitability of VR interventions.
- **Ensure patients have a sufficient degree of general media literacy** (Groeben & Hurrelmann, 2002), such as knowledge about VR technology and its potential side effects.
- **Educate patients on the potential side effects and symptoms** to watch out for during and after VR sessions and prepare them for their VR experiences (Behr et al., 2005).
- **Ensure proper instruction on how to use and adjust the VR equipment** to minimize the risk of motion sickness, eye strain, and discomfort (Chapter 10).
- **Select appropriate VR content** to minimize motion sickness (Chapter 10).
- **Tailor VR experiences to individual patients' physical abilities and limitations** (McCauley & Sharkey, 1992), such as VR content of underwater that accommodates lying positions for patients with tetraplegia.
- **Adjust the intensity of sensory stimuli,** such as brightness, sound volume, or visual effects, to prevent sensory overload or discomfort.
- **Create a dedicated space for VR sessions** that is free from obstacles or tripping hazards.
- **Clear a safe area** for VR sessions, avoiding use in areas that could cause injury through trips, falls, strikes, loss of balance, or other unsafe conditions. The surface seated or standing on should be level, stable, and clear of obstructions.
- **Move the curtain to signal private time** to avoid any disturbances during the session.
- **Ensure that the participants' physical conditions are fit** for maintaining the required posture and movements during VR use (Chapter 10).
- **Ensure the VR device is properly fitted** to optimize comfort and reduce physical strain.

- **Limit the duration of VR usage** to avoid prolonged exposure that may increase the risk of physical discomfort or injury (McCauley & Sharkey, 1992).
- **Prepare to terminate the VR session at any time** if the environment becomes unsafe or the patient experiences physical or emotional discomfort.
- **Maintain hygiene and infection control** through strict compliance with hygiene protocols for VR equipment, including regular disinfection and sterilization procedures (Chapter 10).
- **Use disposable or easily cleanable face masks or covers** for VR headsets to reduce the risk of transmission of infectious diseases (Chapter 10).
- **Continuously evaluate the effectiveness and safety of VR interventions** through patient feedback and ongoing assessment. Follow up after a specified period to assess for long-term negative effects or any residual symptoms (Chapter 10).

Psychological Risks and Recommendations

Despite abundant literature investigating the physical risks associated with VR, limited elaboration is given on psychological risks, particularly in palliative care. It is crucial to recognize that VR experiences may cause emotional distress, which conflicts with the ethical principles of non-maleficence. This section discusses various psychological risk factors and provides recommendations to mitigate them, hoping to alert healthcare professionals to possible psychological adverse effects.

Underlying Maladaptive Cognitions

As VR is found to be an effective tool to induce emotion (Diniz Bernardo et al., 2021), the VR experience can potentially trigger underlying maladaptive cognitions that result in further emotional distress in patients facing end-of-life challenges (Woo & Lee, 2023). The VR experience can evoke memories, fears, or negative thoughts that patients struggle to cope with.

Case Study and Personal Sharing

Mrs. Foxtrot was in her late 60s, receiving palliative care for terminal cancer. She was assessed to have a stable mood prior to VR interventions without significant risk factors that deserve attention. Despite her initial enthusiasm and anticipation for the VR intervention, an unexpected emotional response occurred during the VR experience. As she immersed herself in the serene underwater environment, she suddenly burst into tears. She expressed, "I am useless as a mother as I cannot bring my children to enjoy the sea world like this again," "I am weird as I'm supposed to be happy enjoying such a peaceful environment." I paused the VR exposure and provided her with a safe and supportive space to express her feelings.

Through active listening, I validated her emotions and thoughts, acknowledging the challenges she has been facing in her current situation. I reassured her that her emotional response was understandable, given the complexities of her illness and the impact it had on her self-perception. To facilitate a therapeutic shift in her maladaptive cognitions, I gently explored alternative cognitions by highlighting her inherent worth as a loving mother, independent of her current health condition. I emphasized that experiencing sadness or vulnerability in response to the VR intervention did not diminish her value or make her "weird." Instead, it was a reflection of the intricacies of her emotional journey.

The whole session helped me recognize that VR experience can trigger inner thoughts or emotions easily. It is important to screen out patients who may be vulnerable to such technology. However, there is a possibility that patients experience emotional distress that is unpredictable. Even though VR interventions may trigger maladaptive thinking, I appraise the VR experience as a valuable means to identify a patient's hot cognitions in a short period of time, which paves the way for timely psychological interventions such as cognitive and emotional processing. Though unintended, the VR experience renders a platform for emotional and cognitive work to intervene.

Emotional Vulnerability

Patients under palliative care often experience substantial emotional and existential suffering. Depression is common in the palliative care population, with an estimated prevalence ranging from 24% to 70% (Perusinghe et al., 2021). Anticipatory grief occurs when reacting to the impending loss of life, identity, hopes, and future plans (Cheng et al., 2010; Rando, 2000). As the VR environment is connected closely to the user's perceptual system with high degrees of immersion (Behr et al., 2005), VR may induce intense emotions, which can negatively affect their coping abilities, leading to unfavourable responses (Whitbeck, 1993). For instance, if a user perceives a loss of control in the VR environment, he or she may have an aggressive reaction (Baumeister, 1999). As it is not uncommon to have adjustment reactions at the end-of-life stage, VR interventions, if not carefully tailored, may exacerbate mood problems.

Personal Sharing

In clinical settings, patients with depressive moods often show low motivation for novel interventions such as VR technology. It is understandable, as decreased interest or pleasure in activities is one of the depressive symptoms, as defined by the DSM-5 (American Psychiatric Association, 2013). Invitation for VR technology may trigger responses or cognitions such as, "Nothing can help me now," or "It would not bring any benefits to me." These responses may, to a certain extent, reveal their current coping and adjustment reaction. In view of the depressive mood, it is advised not to deliver VR interventions but other evidence-based interventions such as cognitive behavioral therapy.

Low Degree of Acceptance Towards Palliative Status

Acceptance is one of the five stages of grief suggested by Kübler-Ross (1969). In palliative care, acceptance towards palliative status or impending death has been the therapeutic goal to attain (Zimmermann, 2012). For those who encounter difficulties accepting their current incurable status, VR interventions that aim to virtually bring patients to any preferable places may pose psychological risks. They may inadvertently emphasize the contrast between their unwanted reality and the desired experiences depicted in the virtual world. This contrast can further amplify the sense of demoralization or emotional distress, as VR may unfavourably act as a ruthless reminder of what they can never achieve in real life.

Personal Sharing

In the face of the loss due to terminal illnesses, patients often exhibit a low level of acceptance towards their palliative status. A low level of acceptance is often indicated through expressions such as "Why me?" or "Why do I suffer from the current illness? I have long adopted a healthy lifestyle." When patients still harbour hope for curative treatments, they often show reluctance to engage in interventions that aim at palliative purposes but desire active interventions that can cure their illness. Upon invitation for VR interventions, some of them verbalize sentiments such as, "I remain the same after VR," "It can't help my illness," indicating a belief that such interventions may not help them in whatever ways.

It is, therefore, crucial to recognize that VR interventions may not be applicable to all patients, particularly those who encounter difficulties accepting their incurable status. Acceptance-based psychological interventions may be the prioritized treatment goals rather than those for symptom relief through VR, as the latter may not directly address the profound emotional and existential challenges that they face.

Low Degree of Readiness for Virtual Content

Emergent studies have shown promising results in reminiscence therapy with the help of VR. The immersive nature of VR helps patients review their past in a more immersive way. However, it involves risks of triggering intense emotional responses or unpredictable distress during reminiscence. Without knowing the immersive nature of VR, patients who are not adequately prepared or ready to reminisce about such experiences may be overwhelmed by the vividness and immersiveness of the VR environment, eventually leading to unwanted emotional distress.

Personal Sharing

As a psychologist who has been touched by patients' radiant smiles after VR intervention, I find myself passionate about applying VR interventions to more patients who may benefit from it. However, I always remind myself that not all patients may be ready for a virtual experience, particularly for those who may not want to access the virtual materials that may trigger unpreferable memories. Although VR technology offers a unique opportunity to transport patients across time and place, it is crucial to consider a patient's readiness and willingness to access recollections. As coping strategies differ, not all patients are ready to access past memories. It is, therefore, advisable to conduct a thorough risk and need assessment, especially on the patient's readiness for VR experiences to minimize emotional distress (Chapter 10).

Reentry Problems

Another psychological risk is the unfavourable transition from the virtual to the real-world environment. Patients may find it difficult to adjust to reality once the VR session ends. Such difficulties are labelled as reentry problems (Behr et al., 2005). Reentry problems occur when a user finds it difficult to leave the VR environment, readapt to the real world, or differentiate between virtuality and reality (Behr et al., 2005). These problems may lead to cognitive complications such as confusion when they forget where the source of information is from (Shapiro & Lang, 1991; Appel & Schreier, 2001).

Personal Sharing

I have not encountered patients who presented with significant reentry problems after VR interventions, possibly due to the pre-VR risk assessment and preparation work that may have minimized the associated risks. There has been even a significant portion of patients who request repeated VR sessions. In my opinion, it is important to strike an optimal balance between allowing patients to enjoy the benefits of virtual immersion while avoiding excessive attachment or dependency on the virtual environment. Clinical strategies were delineated in Chapter 10 to facilitate a smooth transition from the virtual to the real world.

Recommendations

1. **Conduct thorough psychological assessments** of each patient's psychological and emotional state before implementing VR interventions (Behr et al., 2005). Consider factors such as history of psychiatric problems, psychological readiness for VR interventions, and degree of acceptance towards their current condition when determining the suitability of VR interventions (Woo & Lee, 2023) (Chapter 10).
2. **Establish clear exclusion criteria** to identify patients who may be at higher risk for experiencing adverse psychological effects from VR (Woo & Lee, 2023) (Chapter 10).
3. **Use screening tools** (Lundin et al., 2023).
4. **Conduct standardized benefit-risk analysis** (Lundin et al., 2023).
5. **Collaborate with the healthcare team** to ensure comprehensive assessment and management of clinical problems such as depressive mood and active psychosis before VR interventions (Chapter 10).
6. **Tailor VR experiences to individual needs** (McCauley & Sharkey, 1992) by conducting needs assessments to identify and prioritize individual requirements (Woo & Lee, 2023).
7. **Select appropriate VR content** that suits individual needs (McCauley & Sharkey, 1992), minimizing the risks of triggering maladaptive cognitions or exacerbating emotional distress (Woo & Lee, 2023).
8. **Instruct patients on the method of termination** in the event of intense or intolerable emotions (Behr et al., 2005).
9. **Prepare to provide immediate psychological support** when needed (Woo & Lee, 2023), ensuring the presence of trained mental health professionals who can offer immediate support and interventions during and after VR sessions.
10. **Monitor and actively listen to patient responses** during VR experiences (Chapter 10).

11. **Provide a structured transition process** from the virtual to the real world, preparing for debriefing and grounding exercises, or relaxation exercises to help patients manage any emotional distress that may arise during or after VR sessions (Chapter 10).

12. **Continuously evaluate the effectiveness and safety of VR interventions** through patient feedback and ongoing assessments. Follow up after a specified period to assess for long-term negative effects or any residual symptoms (Chapter 10).

13. **Stay updated with the latest research and best practices** in using VR in palliative care, particularly on the possible psychological adverse effects, to enhance the quality and safety of interventions (Woo, 2023).

Conclusions

As an emerging and novel therapeutic tool, VR technology appears to offer tremendous opportunities to palliate symptoms and address biopsychosocial-spiritual needs. However, it is essential to be fully aware of the possible adverse effects. This chapter has provided an in-depth exploration of the possible physical and psychological risks of using VR technology in palliative care. Alongside these risks, a comprehensive set of recommendations has been presented, hoping to uphold the ethical principles of *beneficence* and *non-maleficence*. Adhering to ethical standards involves comprehensive training, which will be elaborated in the next chapter. It is hoped that healthcare professionals can strike an optimal balance between optimizing the therapeutic benefits of VR interventions and prioritizing the safety of our vulnerable patients. As VR technology continues to evolve, ongoing research and vigilance are crucial to refine and adapt these recommendations.

References

American Psychiatric Association. (2013). *Diagnostic and statistical manual of mental disorders* (Text Rev., 5th ed.). https://doi.org/10.1176/appi.books.9780890425787

Appel, M., & Schreier, M. (2003, October 9–10). *The role of presence in distinguishing between fact and fiction.* Poster presented at the European Presence Research Conference, Eindhoven, The Netherlands. (Original work published 2001)

Baniasadi, T., Ayyoubzadeh, S. M., & Mohammadzadeh, N. (2020). Challenges and practical considerations in applying virtual reality in medical education and treatment. *Oman Medical Journal, 35*(3), e125.

Baumeister, R. F. (1999). The nature and structure of the self: An overview. In R. F. Baumeister (Ed.), *The self in social psychology* (pp. 1–20). Psychology Press.

Beauchamp, T. L., & Childress, J. F. (2019). *Principles of biomedical ethics* (8th ed.). Oxford University Press.

Behr, K.-M., Nosper, A., Klimmt, C., & Hartmann, T. (2005). Some practical considerations of ethical issues in VR research. *Presence: Teleoperators and Virtual Environment, 14*(6), 668–676. https://doi.org/10.1162/105474605775196535

Botella, C., Pérez-Ara, M. Á., Bretón-López, J., Quero, S., García-Palacios, A., & Baños, R. M. (2016). In vivo versus augmented reality exposure in the treatment of small animal phobia: A randomized controlled trial. *PLoS One, 11*(2), e0148237.

Cheng, J. O. Y., Lo, R. S. K., Chan, F. M. Y., Kwan, B. H. F., & Woo, J. (2010). An exploration of anticipatory grief in advanced cancer patients. *Psycho-Oncology (Chichester, England), 19*(7), 693–700. https://doi.org/10.1002/pon.1613

Diniz Bernardo, P., Bains, A., Westwood, S., & Mograbi, D. C. (2021). Mood induction using virtual reality: A systematic review of recent findings. *Journal of Technology in Behavioral Science, 6*(1), 3–24. https://doi.org/10.1007/s41347-020-00152-9

Edmunds, A., & Morris, A. (2000). The problem of information overload in business organisations: A review of the literature. *International Journal of Information Management, 20*, 17–28.

Fisher, R. S., Acharya, J. N., Baumer, F. M., French, J. A., Parisi, P., Solodar, J. H., Szaflarski, J. P., Thio, L. L., Tolchin, B., Wilkins, A. J., & Kasteleijn-Nolst Trenité, D. (2022). Visually sensitive seizures: An updated review by the epilepsy foundation. *Epilepsia, 63*(4), 739–768.

Groeben, N., & Hurrelmann, B. (Hrsg.). (2002). *Medienkompetenz. Voraussetzungen, Dimensionen, Funktionen [Me media literacy. Conditions, dimensions, functions]*. Juventa.

Han, J., Bae, S. H., & Suk, H. J. (2017). Comparison of visual discomfort and visual fatigue between head-mounted display and smartphone. *Electronic Imaging, 29*, 212–217.

Helmersen, P., Jalalian, A., Moran, G., & Norman, F. (2001). *Impacts of information overload, Eurescom, disponible en ligne*. http://www.eurescom.de/public/projectresults/P900-series/947d1.asp

Horlings, C. G., Van Engelen, B. G., Allum, J. H., & Bloem, B. R. (2008). A weak balance: The contribution of muscle weakness to postural instability and falls. *Nature Clinical Practice Neurology, 4*(9), 504–515.

Kennedy, R. S., Stanney, K. M., & Dunlap, W. P. (2000). Duration and exposure to virtual environments: Sickness curves during and across sessions. *Presence: Teleoperators and Virtual Environments, 9*(5), 463–472.

Kim, E., & Shin, G. (2018). Head rotation and muscle activity when conducting document editing tasks with a head-mounted display. *Proceedings of the Human Factors and Ergonomics Society Annual Meeting, 62*(1), 952–955.

Klapp, O. (1982). Meaning lag in the information society. *Journal of Communication, 32*(2), 56–66.

Kübler-Ross, E. (1969). *On death and dying*. Macmillan.

Levy, F., Leboucher, P., Rautureau, G., Komano, O., Millet, B., & Jouvent, R. (2016). Fear of falling: Efficacy of virtual reality associated with serious games in elderly people. *Neuropsychiatric Disease and Treatment*, 877–881.

Lundin, R. M., Yeap, Y., & Menkes, D. B. (2023). Adverse effects of virtual and augmented reality interventions in psychiatry: Systematic review. *JMIR Mental Health, 10*, e43240. https://doi.org/10.2196/43240

McCauley, M. E., & Sharkey, T. J. (1992). Cybersickness: Perception of self-motion in virtual environments. *Presence: Teleoperators and Virtual Environments, 1*(3), 311–318.

Moore, N., Dempsey, K., Hockey, P., Jain, S., Poronnik, P., Shaban, R. Z., & Ahmadpour, N. (2021). Innovation during a pandemic: Developing a guideline for infection prevention and control to support education through virtual reality. *Frontiers in Digital Health, 3*, 628452.

Penumudi, S. A., Kuppam, V. A., Kim, J. H., & Hwang, J. (2020). The effects of target location on musculoskeletal load, task performance, and subjective discomfort during virtual reality interactions. *Applied ergonomics, 84,* 103010.

Perusinghe, M., Chen, K. Y., & McDermott, B. (2021). Evidence-based management of depression in palliative care: A systematic review. *Journal of Palliative Medicine, 24*(5), 767–781. https://doi.org/10.1089/jpm.2020.0659

Postman, N. (1995). *The end of education: Redefining the value of school* (1st ed.). Knopf.

Rando, T. A. (2000). Anticipatory mourning: A review and critique of the literature. In T. A. Rando (Ed.), *Clinical dimensions of anticipatory mourning: Theory and practice in working with the dying, Their loved ones, and their caregivers.* Research Press.

Riccio, G. E., & Stoffregen, T. A. (1991). An ecological theory of motion sickness and postural instability. *Ecological Psychology, 3*(3), 195–240.

Roberts, S. C., Havill, N. L., Flores, R. M., Hendrix, C. A., II, Williams, M. J., Feinn, R. S., Choi, S. J., Martinello, R. A., Marks, A. M., & Murray, T. S. (2022). Disinfection of virtual reality devices in health care settings: In vitro assessment and survey study. *Journal of Medical Internet Research, 24*(12), e42332.

Rutala, W. A., & Weber, D. J. (2016). Disinfection and sterilization in health care facilities: An overview and current issues. *Infectious Disease Clinics, 30*(3), 609–637.

Schmidt, M., Newbutt, N., Schmidt, C., & Glaser, N. (2021). A process-model for minimizing adverse effects when using head mounted display-based virtual reality for individuals with autism. *Frontiers in Virtual Reality, 2,* 611740.

Shapiro, M. A., & Lang, A. (1991). Making television reality. Unconscious processes in the construction of social reality. *Communication Research, 18*(5), 685–705.

Sheppard, A. L., & Wolffsohn, J. S. (2018). Digital eye strain: Prevalence, measurement and amelioration. *BMJ Open Ophthalmology, 3*(1), e000146.

Smith, S. P., & Burd, E. L. (2019). Response activation and inhibition after exposure to virtual reality. *Array, 3,* 100010.

Souchet, A. D., Philippe, S., Zobel, D., Ober, F., Lévêque, A., & Leroy, L. (2018, November). Eyestrain impacts on learning job interview with a serious game in virtual reality: A randomized double-blinded study. In *Proceedings of the 24th ACM symposium on virtual reality software and technology* (pp. 1–12). https://doi.org/10.1145/3281505.3281509

Szpak, A., Michalski, S. C., Saredakis, D., Chen, C. S., & Loetscher, T. (2019). Beyond feeling sick: The visual and cognitive aftereffects of virtual reality. *IEEE Access, 7,* 130883–130892.

Thye, M. D., Bednarz, H. M., Herringshaw, A. J., Sartin, E. B., & Kana, R. K. (2018). The impact of atypical sensory processing on social impairments in autism spectrum disorder. *Developmental Cognitive Neuroscience, 29,* 151–167.

Van Tulder, M., Malmivaara, A., & Koes, B. (2007). Repetitive strain injury. *The Lancet, 369*(9575), 1815–1822.

Weech, S., Kenny, S., & Barnett-Cowan, M. (2019). Presence and cybersickness in virtual reality are negatively related: A review. *Frontiers in psychology, 10,* 158.

Whitbeck, C. (1993). Virtual environments: Ethical issues and significant confusions. *Presence: Teleoperators and Virtual Environments, 2*(2), 147–152.

Woo, O. K. L. (2023). Integrating knowledge, skills, and attitudes: Professional training required for virtual reality therapists in palliative care. *Frontiers in Medical Technology, 5,* 1268662. https://doi.org/10.3389/fmedt.2023.1268662

Woo, O. K. L., & Lee, A. M. (2023). A perspective on potential psychological risks and solutions of using virtual reality in palliative care. *Frontiers in Virtual Reality*, *4*, 1256641. https://doi.org/10.3389/frvir.2023.1256641

Yan, Y., Chen, K., Xie, Y., Song, Y., & Liu, Y. (2019). The effects of weight on comfort of virtual reality devices. In *Advances in ergonomics in design: Proceedings of the AHFE 2018 international conference on ergonomics in design, July 21–25, 2018, Loews Sapphire Falls Resort at Universal Studios, Orlando, Florida, USA* (pp. 239–248). Springer International Publishing.

Yu, X., Weng, D., Guo, J., Jiang, H., & Bao, Y. (2018, October). Effect of using HMDs for one hour on preteens visual fatigue. In *2018 IEEE international symposium on mixed and augmented reality adjunct (ISMAR-adjunct)* (pp. 93–96). IEEE.

Zhang, Y., Yang, Y., Feng, S., Qi, J., Li, W., & Yu, J. (2020, July 16–20). The evaluation on visual fatigue and comfort between the VR HMD and the iPad. In *Advances in physical, social & occupational ergonomics: Proceedings of the AHFE 2020 virtual conferences on physical ergonomics and human factors, social & occupational ergonomics and cross-cultural decision making, USA* (pp. 213–219). Springer International Publishing.

Zimmermann, C. (2012). Acceptance of dying: A discourse analysis of palliative care literature. *Social Science & Medicine (1982)*, *75*(1), 217–224. https://doi.org/10.1016/j.socscimed.2012.02.047

12 Professional Training in Using Virtual Reality Interventions

Introduction

Imagine a terminally ill patient immersed in the tranquility of a serene beach sunset in the virtual environment, feeling a momentary escape from his suffering reality. Suddenly, the patient bursts into tears, preoccupied with negative emotions that he may not fully understand. In this vulnerable moment, the VR facilitator, untrained in handling such emotional crises, finds himself uncertain and ill-equipped to provide the necessary support, especially with no mental health specialist present. This condition highlights the critical importance of professional training for VR facilitators. While VR equipment is widely accessible and can be technically operated by various individuals, its therapeutic application—especially in clinical contexts like palliative care—demands specific knowledge, skills, and attitudes to ensure quality delivery and ethical practice.

Building on the content of Chapter 11, which addresses the possible adverse effects associated with VR interventions, this chapter emphasizes strategies for minimizing these potential risks to uphold the principles of beneficence and non-maleficence (Beauchamp & Childress, 2019). This chapter is structured into three crucial training aspects: knowledge, skills, and attitudes (Williams, 2016). Each aspect will be elaborated in relation to the three essential roles of clinical, technical, and supervisory in VR facilitation (Table 12.1). The chapter will conclude with a discussion on the importance of a bioethics committee to ensure the ethical implementation of VR interventions. Since there has been limited literature discussing this topic in palliative care settings, the suggested training elaborated in this chapter chiefly draws on my own insights and clinical experiences.

Clinical Knowledge

Delivering VR interventions to patients under palliative care requires VR facilitators to have specific clinical knowledge to ensure optimal care and support.

DOI: 10.4324/9781003518327-17

Table 12.1 The necessary knowledge, skills, and attitude for the clinical, technical, and supervisory role of VR facilitators

	Knowledge	Skills	Attitude
Clinical	• Palliative Care Principles and Specific Needs • Psychological and Therapeutic Knowledge • Research and Evidence-based Practice	• Empathy and Compassion • Effective Communication Skills • Psychological Assessment Skills • Psychological Treatment Skills • Ethical Acumen and Responsibility • Clinical Adaptability and Flexibility	• Non-Judgemental Attitude • Cultural Diversity and Sensitivity
Technical	• Basic Knowledge of VR Equipment and Software • Data Storage and Confidentiality	• VR Equipment and Software Setup • Data Security	• Safety Awareness • Problem-Solving Attitude • Continuous Learning and Adaptation
Supervisory	• Clinical Supervision and Mentoring • Quality Assurance and Evaluation	• Training and Development • Case Management • Communication and Advocacy	• Accountability • Support and Empowerment

Palliative Care Principles and Specific Needs

At the end-of-life stage, patients encounter specific challenges and needs. To ensure that VR intervention caters to their unique needs, VR facilitators require clinical knowledge that relates to the principles and goals of palliative care. This includes the person-centred approach, biopsychosocial-spiritual model, and symptom management (see Chapter 1). Specifically, VR facilitators should be knowledgeable about end-of-life issues, such as existential concerns, anticipatory grief, and coping with dying. It is considered essential as VR facilitators may need to select appropriate VR content to suit individual needs. In addition, some VR software often incorporates this knowledge and approach within VR experiences. It may require clinical acumen for an appropriate judgement on VR content selection to meet individual needs.

Psychological and Therapeutic Knowledge

In the clinical role, it is recommended to have basic knowledge in psychology or related mental health disciplines. This knowledge facilitates psychological assessments such as need and risk assessment, understanding patients' values and preferences, selecting appropriate VR software, and providing psychological support when needed. VR facilitators are also recommended to have good understanding of evidence-based psychological interventions, such as cognitive behavioural therapy, mindfulness-based interventions, and life review interventions. Some VR software may have already incorporated these traditional approaches within VR experiences.

Research and Evidence-based Practice

It is advised to deliver VR interventions which have been studied and supported by research evidence. VR facilitators need to keep abreast of the latest research and evidence-based practices of VR interventions in palliative care. VR facilitators are also recommended to stay updated on literature and emerging guidelines or best practices to ensure quality and ethical delivery.

Technical Knowledge

Most healthcare professionals may not receive prior training on the technical operations of advanced technology. In case of technical problems during VR sessions, the intervention process may be hindered. To maintain basic operation, VR facilitators are required to have basic knowledge of VR systems and hardware equipment. They should be knowledgeable about VR virtual platforms such as various apps, as elaborated on in Chapters 7–9. This includes understanding the available VR resources, their features, and therapeutic goals so that appropriate VR content can be selected to meet individual needs. For ethical practices, VR facilitators should have good data and confidential management, such as secure storage or proper handling of self-recorded VR content.

Supervisory Knowledge

VR facilitators are suggested to process adequate supervisor knowledge in both VR technology and clinical interventions for training aspiring VR facilitators.

Clinical Supervision and Mentoring

Supervisory knowledge refers to expertise in clinical supervision and mentoring in terms of VR interventions. VR supervisors require relevant knowledge to provide professional guidance, support, and development opportunities to the VR team for case discussions and consultations. This can be achieved through conducting regular supervision sessions, holding VR workshops, sharing updated technology, offering constructive feedback, and fostering a positive learning environment. VR supervisors may also consider designing training programs tailored to VR interventions in specific palliative care settings, such as hospices, homes for older adults, and community centres.

Quality Assurance and Evaluation

Supervisory knowledge also refers to the principles of quality assurance and evaluation methods regarding VR interventions in palliative care. Such knowledge aims to ensure that VR interventions is evidence-based with minimal adverse effects. VR supervisors can help achieve quality assurance through monitoring and evaluating patient progress, developing quality assurance processes, and launching program evaluations to ensure the quality of VR interventions.

Clinical Skills

When delivering VR interventions to patients under palliative care, VR facilitators require specific clinical skills to ensure a safe and effective therapeutic intervention.

Empathy and Compassion

Patients under palliative care encounter not only physical and psychological distress but also existential challenges. VR facilitators must possess strong empathetic and compassionate skills to understand the unique needs of individual patients under the person-centred approach (Epstein & Street, 2007; Institute of Medicine, 2001; National Health Priority Action Council, 2006) (see Chapter 1). It implies clinical sensitivity to individual conditions such as pain, coping repertoire, existential distress, and related concerns. VR-assisted intervention should build on a supportive and non-judgmental relationship with the empathic presence of the VR facilitators.

Effective Communication Skills

Effective communication skills are considered essential for VR facilitators. It helps to establish trust, build rapport, and communicate effectively with patients for psychological assessment and progress monitoring. It helps understand patients' goals, preferences, and limitations, allowing for clinical judgement for the appropriate selection of VR content. Effective communication is also needed to collaborate with family members and multidisciplinary palliative care teams, including physicians, nurses, and social workers, to integrate VR interventions into the overall treatment plan in palliative care.

Psychological Assessment Skills

Risk and need assessments prior to VR interventions are recommended to optimize therapeutic benefits (See Chapter 10). Such assessments require clinical skills to assess the suitability of VR interventions for patients. The clinical skills related to performing behavioural observations include reviewing medical records, conducting a patient interview, and collecting collateral information. It involves continuous evaluation of the effectiveness and safety of VR interventions through patient feedback and ongoing assessment. Conducting assessments not only helps determine if VR is appropriate for individual patients but also assesses if any adaptations or modifications are needed, eventually maximizing therapeutic benefits while minimizing possible risks (see Chapter 11). In addition, VR facilitators also need to make clinical judgements on whether traditional psychological interventions or VR interventions would produce better therapeutic benefits to suit the individual patient. Traditional psychological interventions may be more beneficial to some patients, such as those who are less receptive to advanced technology or unready for virtual travelling through VR.

Psychological Treatment Skills

Woo and Lee (2023b), in their perspective paper, recommend psychological interventions following immersive VR exposure. Examples of psychological interventions include psychoeducation (such as educating on the relationship between positive activities and mood improvement), strength-based interventions (such as reinforcing a patient's openness for innovative interventions like VR and active coping), acceptance-based interventions (such as facilitating acceptance towards the uncontrollability and uncertainty in life), cognitive and emotional processing (such as processing anticipatory grief). In addition, emotional distress provoked by VR experience requires immediate delivery of treatment that requires professional skills such as those from counsellors, social workers, or clinical psychologists.

Ethical Acumen and Responsibility

Similar to traditional psychological interventions, the practice of VR interventions must adhere to ethical guidelines and maintain professional standards in palliative care. This includes obtaining informed consent for patients in receiving VR interventions, respecting patient autonomy on trying or not trying VR, and ensuring privacy and confidentiality in terms of the virtual or any other clinical information. VR facilitators should also be mindful of cultural and spiritual considerations that may impact the VR therapeutic outcome.

Clinical Adaptability and Flexibility

Patients at their end-of-life stage may experience fluctuating moods or present with changing needs during their illness journey. VR facilitators need to be sensitive, adaptable, and flexible in adjusting VR interventions to accommodate these changes. For example, facilitators may need to flexibly modify the duration, intensity, or content of the VR experiences to meet individual needs (McCauley & Sharkey, 1992). VR facilitators also need to be sensitive and responsive to any signs of physical or emotional discomfort and provide timely psychological interventions.

Technical Skills

VR facilitators should be skilled in setting up and calibrating VR systems, including headsets, controllers, VR apps, VR cameras, and internet connections. Minimal requirements of technical operations include proper set up for optimal performance and patient comfort. The lack of proper set up may pose risks to patients, such as physical discomforts like dizziness or prolonged VR sessions. Under the person-centred principle, VR facilitators also require skills to select appropriate VR content that matches the individual's values, needs, and preferences. They should also be able to adjust the technical operation to meet specific requirements, such as adjusting visual settings, audio options, and interaction methods, e.g., using remote control or not. To accommodate the needs of patients who are bedbound or have paraplegia, VR technical operations should cater for use while lying down or in a reclined position. Specific skills are also needed to securely handle clinical data and ensure the confidentiality of information.

Supervisory Skills

As VR technology continues to evolve, facilitators must be equipped not only with supervisory and technical knowledge but also with the skills necessary to support aspiring VR facilitators, address concerns, and foster a positive and inclusive atmosphere.

Training and Development

As there is a growing number of patients in need of palliative care worldwide, experienced VR facilitators are responsible for training aspiring VR facilitators to expand the coverage of VR interventions. In addition to aspiring VR facilitators, training can also be rendered to patient assistants or other support staff who can assist in the delivery of VR interventions. Tasks that can be assisted by the support staff include technical set up of the VR equipment, holding the VR headset to decrease subjective weight during VR exposure, and conducting outcome measures. It may allow the VR facilitator to focus on important clinical tasks, such as observing and providing timely feedback to patients during the VR experience.

Case Management

Like traditional psychological interventions, VR facilitators require case management skills to oversee the VR interventions, monitor intervention progress, and ensure that interventions are aligned with the patient's goals and needs. They also need communication skills to discuss with the multi-disciplinary team and family members patient needs, daily functioning, and psychological well-being. In case of emotional distress, VR facilitators need to communicate with other trained professionals, such as counsellors, psychiatrists, or clinical psychologists, for further support.

Communication and Advocacy

Effective communication and advocacy skills are essential for VR facilitators in supervisory roles. Advocacy work includes educating stakeholders on the use of VR in palliative care settings, promoting awareness of VR intervention that is evidence-based, and demonstrating the therapeutic potential of VR interventions through clinical case sharing. In addition, VR facilitators may engage in research projects that serve to validate the efficacy of VR interventions in palliative care. Sharing research results on various occasions, such as interventional conferences and journal publications, may facilitate widespread adoption of such evidenced-based interventions across the globe.

Clinical Attitude

A favourable clinical attitude is essential for VR facilitators to ensure the quality and effectiveness of VR interventions. Not only can a favourable clinical attitude enhance the therapeutic benefits of VR, but also contribute to the overall well-being of patients, ensuring that each interaction is both impactful and compassionate.

Non-Judgemental Attitude

As individuals differ in terms of coping strategies (Lazarus & Folkman, 1984), they have different appraisals or degrees of readiness for the use of VR interventions. VR facilitators require a non-judgemental attitude starting from the moment of inviting their patients to terminating the sessions with feedback received. It is recommended not to make any assumptions or impose personal opinions on patients; for example, assuming that travelling virtually to a favourable destination would surely help patients fulfill their last wishes. Instead, VR facilitators are suggested to provide a supportive and non-judegmental environment for patients to freely express their needs and preferences.

Cultural Diversity and Sensitivity

Patients from clinical settings often come from diverse cultural and religious backgrounds. With different grown-up experiences and cultural backgrounds, VR facilitators should be sensitive to their needs and preferences and respectful towards individual values and beliefs. VR facilitators should have such cultural sensitivity and awareness when approaching patients without imposing their own judgement and values. Particularly when patients are at the end-of-life stage, their existential concerns may be dependent upon their spiritual and cultural values. The careful use of VR technology becomes paramount, particularly when palliative care support extends to support the spiritual needs of patients.

Technical Attitude

A specific technical attitude is crucial for the effective and safe use of VR to ensure seamless and engaging VR experiences for patients. This attitude not only enhances the overall effectiveness of VR interventions but also instills confidence in patients to try novel and innovative interventions.

Safety Awareness

As discussed in Chapter 11 on possible adverse effects of VR interventions, VR interventions may bring harm if not managed well. VR facilitators should have a strong awareness of its possible side effects to avoid any unnecessary harm to patients. With the safety awareness, they are advised to keep abreast of the best practices or relevant guidelines and to take every precaution to minimize harm to patients. VR facilitators should also make accurate documentation and reporting of technical aspects. In case of any technical issues and the necessary adjustments made to suit an individual's needs, such documentation may keep track of patient progress for continual monitoring and help to minimize similar technical issues. VR facilitators should proactively seek technical support whenever necessary to ensure smooth and effective operation.

Problem-Solving Attitude

It is understandable that healthcare professionals are not professionally trained in applied science that may pose challenges for VR operations in palliative care setting. It is also not uncommon to encounter technical issues, such as connection problems, when setting up VR equipment. VR facilitators therefore require an open attitude with a problem-solving mindset. It involves a proactive attitude in identifying and resolving technical problems, troubleshooting errors, and actively seeking relevant support to ensure a smooth VR experience for patients. As the VR headset and camera are now designed for public users in a user-friendly way, VR facilitators with a positive and problem-solving attitude are deemed adequate for its smooth technical operations.

Continuous Learning and Adaptation

VR facilitators require a similar mindset of continuous learning and adaptation, particularly in VR or other advanced technology. As more VR or other XR (extended reality) apps are available in the market that are tailored to the needs of patients under palliative care, VR facilitators are advised to have a positive attitude towards continuous learning. Such a favourable attitude also applies to navigating VR hardware or software that are continuously evolving and upgrading and the research field where VR facilitators can be updated on the latest evidenced-based VR interventions.

Supervisory Attitude

A positive supervisory attitude is vital for training aspiring VR facilitators in palliative care, as it sets the tone for effective leadership and mentorship. A constructive supervisory attitude can inspire confidence in aspiring VR facilitators, promote open communication, and ensure that the next generation of VR facilitators is well-prepared to deliver impactful and compassionate care.

Accountability

As VR technology carries potential risks, VR facilitators should be accountable for both themselves and their team in terms of the quality delivery of VR interventions. VR facilitators need to be responsible for their clinical decisions and judgement on the ethical use of VR interventions. They should take the responsibility of ensuring the VR interventions are delivered in a safe and efficacious way. Supervisors should be ready to provide constructive feedback to the supervisees on their clinical performance and patient progress.

Support and Empowerment

The delivery of technology intervention can be challenging for healthcare professionals without a solid background in technology. Supervisors' attitudes on openness, supportiveness, and respect towards aspiring VR facilitators and assistants become critical. It is recommended that supervisors allow a supportive learning environment that facilitates ongoing professional development and personal growth. Positive feedback, encouragement, or other reinforcement of positive performance are encouraged.

Bioethics Committee

To ensure the ethical and quality delivery of VR-assisted interventions among patients with advanced illnesses, the establishment of a specialized bioethics committee is essential. This committee would play a pivotal role in safeguarding the rights and well-being of this vulnerable population by developing comprehensive VR-related policies, procedures, protocols, or guidelines (PPPGs), educating professionals on ethical principles, and providing necessary resources for ethical decision-making in the delivery of VR interventions. This responds to the significant ethical issue, as highlighted by Moloney et al. (2023) in a scoping review, the lack of PPPGs for the development and implementation of VR interventions. Ideally composed of multidisciplinary experts from relevant fields and patient representatives, the committee would address various ethical concerns, including patient safety, privacy, consent, and adherence to the fundamental principles of biomedical ethics.

Conclusions

This chapter underscores the critical importance of professional training in using VR for therapeutic purposes in palliative care, adhering to the ethical principles of beneficence and non-maleficence. The essential attitudes, knowledge, and skills outlined for clinical, technical, and supervisory roles of qualified VR facilitators are considered vital for its ethical practice. Establishing a dedicated bioethics committee to focus on the specific application of VR among end-of-life patients is proposed. The collaborative efforts of all stakeholders are necessary to safeguard the well-being and rights of patients in palliative care while advancing the responsible use of VR technology. This topic is not only relevant but imperative, as it paves the way for the ongoing development of innovative technologies in long-term palliative care.

References

Beauchamp, T. L., & Childress, J. F. (2019). *Principles of biomedical ethics* (8th ed.). Oxford University Press.

Epstein, R., & Street, R. (2007). *Patient-centred communication in cancer care: Promoting healing and reducing suffering.* National Cancer Institute, NIH Publication.

Institute of Medicine. (2001). *Crossing the quality chasm: A new health system for the 21st century.* National Academy Press.

Lazarus, R. S., & Folkman, S. (1984). *Stress, appraisal and coping.* Springer.

McCauley, M. E., & Sharkey, T. J. (1992). Cybersickness: Perception of self-motion in virtual environments. *Presence: Teleoperators and Virtual Environments, 1*(3), 311–318.

Moloney, M., Doody, O., O'Reilly, M., Lucey, M., Callinan, J., Exton, C., Colreavy, S., O'Mahony, F., Meskell, P., & Coffey, A. (2023). Virtual reality use and patient outcomes in palliative care: A scoping review. *Digital Health, 9,* 20552076231207574. https://doi.org/10.1177/20552076231207574

National Health Priority Action Council. (2006). *National service improvement framework for cancer.* Australian Government Department of Health and Ageing.

Williams, A. M. (2016). Skills, attitudes, and knowledge of effective practitioners. In *Helping relationships with older adults: From theory to practice* (p. 263). SAGE Publications, Incorporated. https://doi.org/10.4135/9781071801239.n9

Section V
Others

This final section discusses future directions, addresses frequently asked questions, and offers clinical resources. Chapter 13 explores the future directions of VR interventions, shedding light on the potential advancements and developments that lie ahead in palliative care. Chapter 14 addresses common questions and concerns when considering or implementing VR interventions. Chapter 15 provides a compilation of clinical resources, hopefully serving as a valuable reference for the clinical use of VR.

DOI: 10.4324/9781003518327-18

13 Future Directions

Introduction

With the growing body of evidence supporting the potential of VR, this chapter explores the exciting future research and clinical directions that advance the field. Key directions of exploration include evaluating the efficacy and effectiveness of VR interventions, tailoring VR applications for diverse sub-populations, and investigating long-term effects and potential risks associated with VR use. The chapter also addresses the possible gender differences, the integration of VR with caregiver support systems, cultural adaptations, and the potential of artificial intelligence to personalize VR experiences. The chapter aims to illuminate the future of VR in palliative care and its capacity to provide meaningful therapeutic benefits.

Efficacy and Effectiveness Studies

Recent meta-analysis and systematic reviews on the use of VR for palliative care consistently report that the quality of evidence was low due to small sample sizes, non-randomization methods, and a lack of a comparator arm (Martin et al., 2022; Mo et al., 2022). Despite the emerging randomized controlled studies in adult (Groninger et al., 2021; Bani Mohammad & Ahmad, 2019; Woo et al., 2024) and paediatric palliative care settings (Wong et al., 2021, 2022), more efficacy studies are called for to determine the therapeutic potentials of VR interventions on various aspects of palliative care. Research studies are encouraged to compare the use of VR with other complementary therapies (Bani Mohammad & Ahmad, 2019). The cost-effectiveness and scalability of VR interventions in palliative care is worthy of investigations as well. Pointed out by Moutogiannis et al. (2023) in their rapid review, the direct and indirect costs associated with VR such as connectivity and staff training has been rarely discussed. The economic cost and impact of delivering VR interventions appear to be one future research direction.

DOI: 10.4324/9781003518327-19

Adaptations in Sub-Populations

While empirical studies have increasingly supported the use of VR interventions in palliative care, research focusing on specific sub-populations within this field remains limited. It resonates with Mackey et al. (2020), who highlight future directions for expanding the scope of VR applications in palliative care. VR appears to have therapeutic potential among individuals across different developmental stages facing life-limiting illnesses, such as children, older adults, and individuals with specific medical conditions. This underscores the importance of developing personalized, age-appropriate VR content that addresses the distinct requirements of various sub-populations within palliative care.

Paediatric Palliative Care

The application of VR in palliative care originally targets the adult population, with limited investigations among children or adolescents. However, there is an emergent discussion and studies. The case report from Weingarten et al. (2020) acknowledges the significant potential for VR in paediatric palliative care. The authors advocate its substantial potential for a guided therapy modality to engage young people and identify their priorities, hopes, and goals. An exploratory trial (Wong et al., 2022) shows the potential effectiveness, feasibility, and acceptability of immersive virtual reality for managing anxiety and acute nausea amongst paediatric patients with cancer. Results of another randomized controlled trial conducted led by the same principal investigator (Wong et al., 2021) support the safe and effective use of VR for pain and anxiety management among paediatric cancer patients undergoing peripheral intravenous cannulation procedures.

As VR content can incorporate interactive and engaging elements such as animated characters or gamified activities, VR interventions appear to be appealing to the younger generations. A study has shown that immersion in a VR environment can help redirect attention among paediatric patients, reducing their anxiety and pain during medical procedures (Arane et al., 2017). The unlimited potential of its application in paediatric care sheds light on future research and clinical directions.

Geriatric Palliative Care

A meta-analysis study has provided supportive evidence for the use of VR in geriatric populations in terms of improving functional mobility (Corregidor-Sánchez et al., 2021), ameliorating frailty and fall risks (Lee et al., 2023), improving cognitive function (Yan et al., 2022) and physical functions (Ren et al., 2023). The findings shed light on its potential in rehabilitation among older adults in palliative care settings. However, research that specifically targets the use of VR in geriatric palliative care is scarce. More investigations on the VR interventions that cater to the specific needs of this population are recommended.

Specific Medical Conditions

Most research studies on the VR application in palliative care settings appear to target patients with cancer or patients under palliative care in general; there is a scarcity of investigations that target sub-population groups with specific medical conditions. This section explores the potential of VR intervention in patients with heart failure, chronic obstructive pulmonary disease, cord compression, cognitive impairments, and other needs.

Heart Failure

Advanced technology has been explored to support patients with heart failure (Mohebali & Kittleson, 2021). VR, in particular, can include immersive educational modules that help patients understand their condition, manage medications, and adopt healthy lifestyle choices. For example, Kieu et al. (2023) use a VR platform to educate patients with congenital heart diseases about their illness and treatment options, which is found to be feasible, enjoyable and helpful in learning about the disease. Groninger et al. (2021) report that participants with advanced heart failure from the VR experimental group experience a 1.5 unit comparatively greater reduction in pain score compared to those in the control group with guided imagery, indicating the potential of VR as an effective nonpharmacologic adjuvant pain management intervention. The authors suggest future studies on the impact of VR therapies on the aspects of illness experience and quality of life other than pain.

Chronic Obstructive Pulmonary Disease

VR interventions appear to hold significant potential for patients with chronic obstructive pulmonary disease (COPD). VR experiences are shown to offer virtual pulmonary rehabilitation exercises, breathing techniques, and education on managing COPD symptoms (Colombo et al., 2022; Rutkowski et al., 2020). Through simulating different environments and altitudes, VR can help patients gradually adapt to various levels of physical exertion and improve their respiratory function, while patients can receive timely feedback on their performances (Colombo et al., 2022). Furthermore, VR interventions can provide psychological support by offering relaxation exercises and distraction therapy and fostering a sense of control and empowerment for individuals living with COPD (Pancini et al., 2023). Its application in patients with COPD in a palliative care setting requires more future investigations.

Cord Compression

Limited studies have investigated the use of VR to address the unique challenges faced by patients with cord compression in palliative care. However, VR appears to be a potential tool in light of its immersive nature and sense of presence. Through virtual environments that simulate safe and engaging exercises, growing evidence from clinical studies shows that VR training improves the neurological function of patients with spinal cord injury, cerebral palsy, and other neurological impairments (Mao et al., 2014). In light of the scientific evidence on its efficacy in pain management (Malloy & Milling, 2010), VR appears to have the potential therapeutic benefit for patients with cord compression that warrants further clinical or research investigations.

Clinical Mood Conditions

As elaborated on in Chapter 3, mood problems have been one of the unmet psychological needs among patients under palliative care. Various studies highlight the prevalence of depression (Miovic & Block, 2007; Mitchell et al., 2011) and anxiety (Sewtz et al., 2021; Wang et al., 2018) in palliative care, thus calling for non-pharmacological approaches (Atkin et al., 2017; Noorani & Montagnini, 2007; Perusinghe et al., 2021). As emerging evidence points to the potential of VR in improving mood (Mo et al., 2022; Moscato et al., 2021), the use of VR in treating clinical mood problems remains a worthwhile area of investigation. For instance, more investigations can focus on the use of VR in supporting cognitive behavioural therapy (Bernatchez et al., 2019) or mindfulness-based stress reduction therapy (Poletti et al., 2019) in palliative care settings. In addition, the use of VR targeting clinical sleep problems, which has been one of the unmet needs in palliative cases (see Chapter 3), may be another promising research area.

Long-term Impact

While most of the acceptance and feasibility of VR interventions in palliative care settings are well established as a single session, its longitudinal impact is yet to be examined (Moutogiannis et al., 2023). A meta-analysis by Wu et al. (2023) has shown that VR interventions are effective in reducing physical and psychological symptoms among cancer patients. However, the author suggests further research with longer follow-up periods to understand the treatment gains over time. The author of a newly developed VR relaxation intervention suggests further investigations on the long-term effect or skill development, such as continual relaxation practice during rehabilitation (Woo & Lee, 2023a). Similarly, Bani Mohammad and Ahmad (2019) propose qualitative exploration into the long-term impact of VR interventions on pain and anxiety. Although the lifespan of a patient is limited, it appears worthy to explore whether the effects of VR interventions can be sustained throughout the rehabilitation journey (Tan et al., 2013; Niki et al., 2019).

Potential Risks

A systematic review by Martin et al. (2022) highlights a few adverse effects associated with VR interventions in palliative care setting, which include claustrophobia (Brungardt et al., 2020), an increase in pain (Ferguson et al., 2020), crying and hallucinations (Ferguson et al., 2020), sore shoulders (Johnson et al., 2020), and visual hallucinations (Albani et al., 2015). In a VR study involving patients with advanced dementia, one participant is found staring at a blank display without the ability to inform the research team (Ferguson et al., 2020). A perspective paper written by Woo and Lee (2023b) highlights three potential psychological conditions that may trigger emotional distress when maladaptive cognitions triggered by the virtual experience are not appropriately processed; when there is a lack of smooth transition from virtual to the real world; and when patients are not psychologically ready for the virtual environment. Future investigations are needed to further investigate the potential psychological risks of using VR in such vulnerable population.

Gender Differences

There has been some research investigating the effect of gender on the experience and acceptance of VR. For instance, a latent sexism is applied in the design of head-mounted display technology in favouring male head physiognomy over female, which makes the technology more comfortable for men than for women (Grassini & Laumann, 2020). Some studies convergently report that women experience motion sickness more than men (MacArthur et al., 2021; Stanney et al., 2020). LaViola (2000) relates the increased chance of motion sickness to women's wider field of view and hormonal changes. In a randomized controlled trial with an adequate sample size, a high female-to-male ratio (70%–30%) is reported in the recruited participants (Woo et al., 2024). The investigators clinically observe that males show higher rates of rejection towards research participation. Further investigations are needed to investigate gender differences, especially in palliative care settings, to ensure the ethical and quality delivery of VR interventions.

VR and Caregivers

A rapid review by Moutogiannis et al. (2023) highlights that the role of VR intervention for caregivers, particularly in reducing burnout, fatigue, and other stress symptoms, has been rarely discussed. Moreover, there have been emerging pilot and feasibility studies focusing on VR-based bereavement support for family members or significant others (Botella et al., 2008; Knowles et al., 2017; Liao et al., 2023; Quero et al., 2019). Despite the preliminary evidence supporting its therapeutic benefits, Pizzoli et al. (2023) critically analyze the possible side-effects as the VR experience with virtual avatars can be extremely emotional when interacting with the lost person. The authors continually raise ethical concerns, such as additional emotional distress and vulnerability posed by the VR experiences. Further investigations on the specific benefits and guidelines for VR interventions on bereavement support and the associated side-effects are essential to ensure ethical practice.

Adaptations Across Culture

In terms of cultural sensitivity and appropriateness, it is essential to understand and respect cultural norms, beliefs, and practices related to illness and death (Cain et al., 2018). VR content, as an advanced technology, should be designed to align with the cultural preferences and values of palliative care patients from diverse backgrounds (Ferguson et al., 2020; Okoro et al., 2024). However, limited studies have adapted the virtual environments to the sociocultural context of different groups, especially when generic foreign VR environments are used that do not resemble local settings (Emmelkamp & Meyerbröker, 2021). It is speculated in the same study that including culturally relevant elements in virtual environments might increase the effectiveness of the treatment by creating a sense of familiarity and a greater sensation of presence among patients. VR interventions should also explore the inclusion of culturally significant elements, such as specific cultural settings, rituals, or spiritual practices (Desselle et al., 2023). Translations in different languages and adapting visual and audio elements to align with cultural aesthetics and preferences are also considered essential (Okoro et al., 2024). Engaging healthcare professionals, patients, families, and cultural experts in the development and evaluation of culturally sensitive VR interventions can provide valuable insights and perspectives (Carr, 2020). Lastly, conducting cross-cultural research studies is advocated to understand the effectiveness and acceptability of VR interventions across cultural settings (Koç & Kafa, 2019). Future investigations can consider comparative studies that explore the similarities and differences in patient experiences, outcomes, and preferences across cultures.

Incorporation of Artificial Intelligence

As technology continues to advance, the integration of artificial intelligence (AI) and robotics holds potential for enhancing VR interventions in palliative care. For instance, AI can be utilized to develop intelligent adaptive VR systems that dynamically adjust the virtual environment and content based on real-time patient data and feedback. AI algorithms can optimize the VR experience by personalizing it to individual needs, providing adaptive content and feedback (Zahabi & Abdul Razak, 2020). It can also enhance sensing and monitoring capabilities, such as using wearable devices or sensors to collect real-time physiological data, including heart rate, respiratory rate, or skin conductance (Kim et al., 2021).

Ethical Considerations

Ethical considerations have been a crucial theme in the use of VR in palliative care. A systematic review and meta-analysis conducted by Mo et al. (2022) advocate the appropriate policy measures to ensure that VR platforms and experiences are monitored for quality. A scoping review by Moloney et al. (2023) concludes that there has been no reports of pre-existing policies, procedures, protocols, or guidelines (PPPGs) used in relation to the design, development, or implementation of VR experiences in palliative care settings. The authors further highlight that several studies have positioned VR as a "therapeutic intervention," which implies it is an evidence-based practice that needs to be facilitated by an intervention specialist or therapist. However, only a few studies have involved a VR specialist that warrant attention (Lloyd & Haraldsdottir, 2021; Woo et al., 2024). Future research should focus on exploring ethical guidelines for VR use, including issues related to patient autonomy, privacy, informed consent, and potential psychological risks (Woo & Lee, 2023b). Robust protocols are also suggested for detecting and reporting adverse reactions in VR research (Lundin et al., 2023). Lastly, future research is advised on professional training for the delivery of VR (Martin et al., 2022; Perna et al., 2021; Woo & Lee, 2023b). Clear ethical frameworks and professional training are required to facilitate responsible and ethical implementation of VR in palliative care settings.

Conclusions

This chapter discusses future research and clinical directions of VR interventions concerning its efficacy and effectiveness, the adaptation for diverse sub-populations, the exploration of long-term impacts and potential risks, the examination of gender differences, the integration of VR with caregiver support, cultural adaptations, and the incorporation of artificial intelligence. Given that VR has emerged as a helpful therapeutic tool in palliative care, further investigations are essential to ensure ethical delivery tailored to the specific needs of this vulnerable population.

References

Albani, G., Pedroli, E., Cipresso, P., Bulla, D., Cimolin, V., Thomas, A. M., Mauro, A., & Riva, G. (2015). Visual hallucinations as incidental negative effects of virtual reality on parkinson's disease patients: A link with neurodegeneration? *Parkinson's Disease, 2015*, 194629.

Arane, K., Behboudi, A., & Goldman, R. D. (2017). VR for pain and anxiety management in children. *Canadian Family Physician, 63*(12), 932–934.

Atkin, N., Vickerstaff, V., & Candy, B. (2017). "Worried to death": The assessment and management of anxiety in patients with advanced life-limiting disease, a national survey of palliative medicine physicians. *BMC Palliative Care, 16*(1), 69. https://doi.org/10.1186/s12904-017-0245-5

Bani Mohammad, E., & Ahmad, M. (2019). Virtual reality as a distraction technique for pain and anxiety among patients with breast cancer: A randomized control trial. *Palliative & Supportive Care, 17*(1), 29–34. https://doi.org/10.1017/S1478951518000639

Bernatchez, M. S., Savard, J., Savard, M.-H., & Aubin, M. (2019). Feasibility of a cognitive-behavioral and environmental intervention for sleep-wake difficulties in community-dwelling cancer patients receiving palliative care. *Cancer Nursing, 42*(5), 396–409. https://doi.org/10.1097/NCC.0000000000000603

Botella, C., Osma, J., Palacios, A. G., Guillén, V., & Baños, R. (2008). Treatment of complicated grief using virtual reality: A case report. *Death Studies, 32*(7), 674–692. https://doi.org/10.1080/07481180802231319

Brungardt, A., Wibben, A., Tompkins, A. F., Shanbhag, P., Coats, H., LaGasse, A. B., Boeldt, D., Youngwerth, J., Kutner, J. S., & Lum, H. D. (2021). Virtual reality-based music therapy in palliative care: A pilot implementation trial. *Journal of Palliative Medicine, 24*(5), 736–742. https://doi.org/10.1089/jpm.2020.0403

Cain, C. L., Surbone, A., Elk, R., & Kagawa-Singer, M. (2018). Culture and palliative care: Preferences, communication, meaning, and mutual decision making. *Journal of Pain and Symptom Management, 55*(5), 1408–1419.

Carr, S. (2020). 'AI gone mental': Engagement and ethics in data-driven technology for mental health. *Journal of Mental Health, 29*(2), 125–130.

Colombo, V., Aliverti, A., & Sacco, M. (2022). VR for COPD rehabilitation: A technological perspective. *Pulmonology, 28*(2), 119–133.

Corregidor-Sánchez, A. I., Segura-Fragoso, A., Rodríguez-Hernández, M., Jiménez-Rojas, C., Polonio-López, B., & Criado-Álvarez, J. J. (2021). Effectiveness of virtual reality technology on functional mobility of older adults: Systematic review and meta-analysis. *Age and Ageing, 50*(2), 370–379. https://doi.org/10.1093/ageing/afaa197

Desselle, M. R., Holland, L. R., McKittrick, A., Kennedy, G., Yates, P., & Brown, J. (2023). "A wanderer's tale": The development of a VR application for pain and quality of life in Australian burns and oncology patients. *Palliative & Supportive Care, 21*(3), 454–460.

Emmelkamp, P. M., & Meyerbröker, K. (2021). VR therapy in mental health. *Annual Review of Clinical Psychology, 17*, 495–519.

Ferguson, C., Shade, M. Y., Blaskewicz Boron, J., Lyden, E., & Manley, N. A. (2020). Virtual reality for therapeutic recreation in dementia hospice care: A feasibility study. *American Journal of Hospice & Palliative Medicine, 37*(10), 809–815. https://doi.org/10.1177/1049909120901525

Grassini, S., & Laumann, K. (2020). Are modern head-mounted displays sexist? A systematic review on gender differences in HMD-mediated virtual reality. *Frontiers in Psychology, 11*, 1604. https://doi.org/10.3389/fpsyg.2020.01604

Groninger, H., Stewart, D., Fisher, J. M., Tefera, E., Cowgill, J., & Mete, M. (2021). Virtual reality for pain management in advanced heart failure: A randomized controlled study. *Palliative Medicine, 35*(10), 2008–2016. https://doi.org/10.1177/02692163211041273

Johnson, T., Bauler, L., Vos, D., Hifko, A., Garg, P., Ahmed, M., & Raphelson, M. (2020). Virtual reality use for symptom management in palliative care: A pilot study to assess user perceptions. *Journal of Palliative Medicine, 23*(9), 1233–1238. https://doi.org/10.1089/jpm.2019.0411

Kieu, V., Sumski, C., Cohen, S., Reinhardt, E., Axelrod, D. M., & Handler, S. S. (2023). The use of VR learning on transition education in adolescents with congenital heart disease. *Pediatric Cardiology, 44*(8), 1856–1860.

Kim, H., Kwon, Y. T., Lim, H. R., Kim, J. H., Kim, Y. S., & Yeo, W. H. (2021). Recent advances in wearable sensors and integrated functional devices for virtual and augmented reality applications. *Advanced Functional Materials, 31*(39), 2005692.

Knowles, L. M., Stelzer, E.-M., Jovel, K. S., & O'Connor, M.-F. (2017). A pilot study of virtual support for grief: Feasibility, acceptability, and preliminary outcomes. *Computers in Human Behavior, 73*, 650–658. https://doi.org/10.1016/j.chb.2017.04.005

Koç, V., & Kafa, G. (2019). Cross-cultural research on psychotherapy: The need for a change. *Journal of Cross-Cultural Psychology, 50*(1), 100–115.

LaViola, J. J. (2000). A discussion of cybersickness in virtual environments. *SIGCHI Bulletin, 32*(1), 47–56. https://doi.org/10.1145/333329.333344

Lee, Y.-H., Lin, C.-H., Wu, W.-R., Chiu, H.-Y., & Huang, H.-C. (2023). Virtual reality exercise programs ameliorate frailty and fall risks in older adults: A meta-analysis. *Journal of the American Geriatrics Society (JAGS), 71*(9), 2946–2955. https://doi.org/10.1111/jgs.18398

Liao, D., Xia, Y., Xu, M., & Ding, M. (2023). A grief farewell scene design for children based on virtual reality. In *International conference on artificial intelligence and industrial design (AIID 2022)* (Vol. 12612, p. 126120G). https://doi.org/10.1117/12.2673048

Lloyd, A., & Haraldsdottir, E. (2021). Virtual reality in hospice: Improved patient well-being. *BMJ Supportive & Palliative Care, 11*(3), 344–350. https://doi.org/10.1136/bmjspcare-2021-003173

Lundin, R. M., Yeap, Y., & Menkes, D. B. (2023). Adverse effects of virtual and augmented reality interventions in psychiatry: Systematic review. *JMIR Mental Health, 10*, e43240. https://doi.org/10.2196/43240

MacArthur, C., Grinberg, A., Harley, D., & Hancock, M. (2021). You're making me sick: A systematic review of how virtual reality research considers gender & cybersickness. In *Proceedings of the 2021 CHI conference on human factors in computing systems* (Article 401, pp. 1–15). Association for Computing Machinery. https://doi.org/10.1145/3411764.3445701

Mackey, B., Bremner, P., & Giuliani, M. (2020). Immersive control of a robot surrogate for users in palliative care. In *Companion of the 2020 ACM/IEEE international conference on human-robot interaction* (pp. 585–587). https://doi.org/10.1145/3371382.3377445

Malloy, K. M., & Milling, L. S. (2010). The effectiveness of VR distraction for pain reduction: A systematic review. *Clinical Psychology Review, 30*(8), 1011–1018.

Mao, Y., Chen, P., Li, L., & Huang, D. (2014). VR training improves balance function. *Neural Regeneration Research, 9*(17), 1628–1634.

Martin, J. L., Saredakis, D., Hutchinson, A. D., Crawford, G. B., & Loetscher, T. (2022). Virtual reality in palliative care: A systematic review. *Healthcare (Basel), 10*(7), 1222.

Miovic, M., & Block, S. (2007). Psychiatric disorders in advanced cancer. *Cancer, 110*(8), 1665–1676. https://doi.org/10.1002/cncr.22980

Mitchell, A. J., Chan, M., Bhatti, H., Halton, M., Grassi, L., Johansen, C., & Meader, N. (2011). Prevalence of depression, anxiety, and adjustment disorder in oncological, haematological, and palliative-care settings: A meta-analysis of 94 interview-based studies. *The Lancet Oncology, 12*(2), 160–174. https://doi.org/10.1016/S1470-2045(11)70002-X

Mo, J., Vickerstaff, V., Minton, O., Tavabie, S., Taubert, M., Stone, P., & White, N. (2022). How effective is VR technology in palliative care? A systematic review and meta-analysis. *Palliative Medicine, 36*(7), 1047–1058.

Mohebali, D., & Kittleson, M. M. (2021). Remote monitoring in heart failure: Current and emerging technologies in the context of the pandemic. *Heart,* 366–372.

Moloney, M., Doody, O., O'Reilly, M., Lucey, M., Callinan, J., Exton, C., Colreavy, S., O'Mahony, F., Meskell, P., & Coffey, A. (2023). Virtual reality use and patient outcomes in palliative care: A scoping review. *Digital Health, 9,* 20552076231207576. https://doi.org/10.1177/20552076231207574

Moscato, S., Sichi, V., Giannelli, A., Palumbo, P., Ostan, R., & Chiari, L. (2021). Virtual reality in home palliative care: Brief report on the effect on cancer-related symptomatology. *Frontiers in Psychology, 12,* 709154.

Moutogiannis, P. P., Thrift, J., Pope, J. K., Browning, M. H. E. M., McAnirlin, O., & Fasolino, T. (2023). A rapid review of the role of virtual reality in care delivery of palliative care and hospice. *Journal of Hospice and Palliative Nursing, 25*(6), 300–308. https://doi.org/10.1097/NJH.0000000000000983

Niki, K., Okamoto, Y., Maeda, I., Mori, I., Ishii, R., Matsuda, Y., Takagi, T., & Uejima, E. (2019). A novel palliative care approach using virtual reality for improving various symptoms of terminal cancer patients: A preliminary prospective, multicenter study. *Journal of Palliative Medicine, 22*(6), 702–707. https://doi.org/10.1089/jpm.2018.0527

Noorani, N. H., & Montagnini, M. (2007). Recognizing depression in palliative care patients. *Journal of Palliative Medicine, 10*(2), 458–464. https://doi.org/10.1089/jpm.2006.0099

Okoro, Y. O., Ayo-Farai, O., Maduka, C. P., Okongwu, C. C., & Sodamade, O. T. (2024). The role of technology in enhancing mental health advocacy: A systematic review. *International Journal of Applied Research in Social Sciences, 6*(1), 37–50.

Pancini, E., Villani, D., & Riva, G. (2023). oVeRcomING COPD: VR and savoring to promote the well-being of patients with chronic obstructive pulmonary disease. *Cyberpsychology, Behavior and Social Networking, 26*(1), 65–67.

Perna, L., Lund, S., White, N., & Minton, O. (2021). The potential of personalized virtual reality in palliative care: A feasibility trial. *American Journal of Hospice and Palliative Medicine®, 38*(12), 1488–1494.

Perusinghe, M., Chen, K. Y., & McDermott, B. (2021). Evidence-based management of depression in palliative care: A systematic review. *Journal of Palliative Medicine, 24*(5), 767–781. https://doi.org/10.1089/jpm.2020.0659

Pizzoli, S. F. M., Monzani, D., Vergani, L., Sanchini, V., & Mazzocco, K. (2023). From virtual to real healing: A critical overview of the therapeutic use of virtual reality to cope with mourning. *Current Psychology (New Brunswick, N.J.)*, *42*(11), 8697–8704. https://doi.org/10.1007/s12144-021-02158-9

Poletti, S., Razzini, G., Ferrari, R., Ricchieri, M. P., Spedicato, G. A., Pasqualini, A., Buzzega, C., Artioli, F., Petropulacos, K., Luppi, M., & Bandieri, E. (2019). Mindfulness-based stress reduction in early palliative care for people with metastatic cancer: A mixed-method study. *Complementary Therapies in Medicine*, *47*, 102218. https://doi.org/10.1016/j.ctim.2019.102218

Quero, S., Molés, M., Campos, D., Andreu-Mateu, S., Baños, R. M., & Botella, C. (2019). An adaptive virtual reality system for the treatment of adjustment disorder and complicated grief: 1-year follow-up efficacy data. *Clinical Psychology and Psychotherapy*, *26*(2), 204–217. https://doi.org/10.1002/cpp.2342

Ren, Y., Lin, C., Zhou, Q., Yingyuan, Z., Wang, G., & Lu, A. (2023). Effectiveness of virtual reality games in improving physical function, balance and reducing falls in balance-impaired older adults: A systematic review and meta-analysis. *Archives of Gerontology and Geriatrics*, *108*, 104924. https://doi.org/10.1016/j.archger.2023.104924

Rutkowski, S., Rutkowska, A., Kiper, P., Jastrzebski, D., Racheniuk, H., Turolla, A., Szczegielniak, J., & Casaburi, R. (2020). VR rehabilitation in patients with chronic obstructive pulmonary disease: A randomized controlled trial. *International Journal of Chronic Obstructive Pulmonary Disease*, 117–124.

Sewtz, C., Muscheites, W., Grosse-Thie, C., Kriesen, U., Leithaeuser, M., Glaeser, D., Hansen, P., Kundt, G., Fuellen, G., & Junghanss, C. (2021). Longitudinal observation of anxiety and depression among palliative care cancer patients. *Annals of Palliative Medicine*, *10*(4), 3836–3846. https://doi.org/10.21037/apm-20-1346

Stanney, K., Fidopiastis, C., & Foster, L. (2020). Virtual reality is sexist: But it does not have to be. *Frontiers in Robotics and AI*, *7*, 4. https://doi.org/10.3389/frobt.2020.00004

Tan, A., Ross, S. P., & Duerksen, K. (2013). Death is not always a failure: Outcomes from implementing an online virtual patient clinical case in palliative care for family medicine clerkship. *Medical Education Online*, *18*(1), 22711. https://doi.org/10.3402/meo.v18i0.22711

Wang, T., Molassiotis, A., Chung, B. P. M., & Tan, J.-Y. (2018). Unmet care needs of advanced cancer patients and their informal caregivers: A systematic review. *BMC Palliative Care*, *17*(1), 96. https://doi.org/10.1186/s12904-018-0346-9

Weingarten, K., Macapagal, F., & Parker, D. (2020). Virtual reality: Endless potential in pediatric palliative care: A case report. *Journal of Palliative Medicine*, *23*(1), 147–149.

Wong, C. L., Li, C. K., Chan, C. W. H., Choi, K. C., Chen, J., Yeung, M. T., & Chan, O. N. (2021). Virtual reality intervention targeting pain and anxiety among pediatric cancer patients undergoing peripheral intravenous cannulation: A randomized controlled trial. *Cancer Nursing*, *44*(6), 435–442. https://doi.org/10.1097/NCC.0000000000000844

Wong, C. L., Li, C. K., Choi, K. C., Wei So, W. K., Yan Kwok, J. Y., Cheung, Y. T., & Chan, C. W. H. (2022). Effects of immersive virtual reality for managing anxiety, nausea and vomiting among paediatric cancer patients receiving their first chemotherapy: An exploratory randomised controlled trial. *European Journal of Oncology Nursing: The Official Journal of European Oncology Nursing Society*, *61*, 102233. https://doi.org/10.1016/j.ejon.2022.102233

Woo, O. K. L., & Lee, A. M. (2023a). Case report: Therapeutic potential of flourishing-life-of-wish VR therapy on relaxation (FLOW-VRT-relaxation)—a novel personalized relaxation in palliative care. *Frontiers in Digital Health, 5,* 1228781.

Woo, O. K. L., & Lee, A. M. (2023b). A perspective on potential psychological risks and solutions of using VR in palliative care. *Frontiers in VR, 4,* https://doi.org/10.3389/frvir.2023.1256641

Woo, O. K. L., Lee, A. M., Ng, R., Eckhoff, D., Lo, R., & Cassinelli, A. (2024). Flourishing-life-of-wish virtual reality relaxation therapy (FLOW-VRT-relaxation) outperforms traditional relaxation therapy in palliative care: Results from a randomized controlled trial. *Frontiers in Virtual Reality, 4.* https://doi.org/10.3389/frvir.2023.1304155

Wu, Y., Wang, N., Zhang, H., Sun, X., Wang, Y., & Zhang, Y. (2023). Effectiveness of VR in symptom management of cancer patients: A systematic review and meta-analysis. *Journal of Pain and Symptom Management, 65*(5), e467–e482.

Yan, M., Zhao, Y., Meng, Q., Wang, S., Ding, Y., Liu, Q., Yin, H., & Chen, L. (2022). Effects of virtual reality combined cognitive and physical interventions on cognitive function in older adults with mild cognitive impairment: A systematic review and meta-analysis. *Ageing Research Reviews, 81,* 101708. https://doi.org/10.1016/j.arr.2022.101708

Zahabi, M., & Abdul Razak, A. M. (2020). Adaptive VR-based training: A systematic literature review and framework. *VR, 24,* 725–752.

14 Frequently Asked Questions

What Patient Groups and in What Context Has VR Been Applied?

VR studies have focused on both adults and children receiving palliative care, whether in hospice facilities or at home (see Chapter 5).

Can VR be Applied to Paediatric Palliative Care?

Primary studies on the use of VR in palliative care are on adult populations, while there are emerging studies investigating its application in children under palliative care. A case report from Weingarten et al. (2020) advocates the potential of VR interventions in paediatric palliative care, while a randomized controlled trial conducted by Wong et al. (2021) indicates that VR is safe and effective in alleviating pain and anxiety among paediatric cancer patients undergoing peripheral intravenous cannulation procedures.

How Long Is the VR Duration Most Recommendable?

Perna et al. (2021) report adopting a flexible duration of VR intervention depending on patients' physical conditions and psychological needs. A systematic review and meta-analysis conducted by Saredakis et al. (2020) highlights that prolonged exposure to VR scenes might be a risk factor for the development of cybersickness.

What Types of VR Experiences Should I Offer to My Patients Under Palliative Care?

The use of VR is advised to follow the palliative care principles such as person-centred and biopsychosocial-spiritual models (see Chapter 1). To align with these principles, it is suggested to conduct a need assessment to identify needs and select VR experiences based on individual preferences (see Chapter 10).

DOI: 10.4324/9781003518327-20

How Can I Integrate VR Interventions Into My Palliative Care Practice?

To integrate VR interventions into palliative care, start by assessing patient needs in your own setting, gathering support from your department for the purchase of relevant equipment, and presenting evidence of VR benefits. Study the potential benefits and risks of VR interventions through updated research, choose user-friendly VR equipment, and organize training for healthcare professionals.

Are There Other Ethical Considerations (Apart From Chapters 11 and 12) When Using VR Interventions in Palliative Care?

Ethical considerations also include the informed consent procedures, patient autonomy, privacy and confidentiality, and the need for ongoing ethical oversight when implementing VR interventions.

Are There Any Ethical Principles Related to Conducting VR Research in Palliative Care?

Conducting VR research in palliative care should follow principles under biomedical ethics (Beauchamp & Childress, 2019), including beneficence, non-maleficence, autonomy, and justice.

What Are the Potential Risks or Side Effects of VR Interventions?

Physical side effects include cybersickness, while psychological adverse effects include heightened emotional distress (see Chapter 11).

What Are the Costs Involved in Using VR in a Palliative Care Setting?

Costs involve the purchase of VR hardware and software. VR equipment includes the VR headset with remotes and VR camera (see Chapter 10), while the software includes the VR applications or programs. There are freely available VR applications which have been validated by research (see Section III).

How Can I Measure the Efficacy of VR Interventions for My Patients?

Healthcare professionals may use outcome measures or assessment tools to evaluate the efficacy of VR interventions for patients under palliative care, monitor patient progress, and document changes in physical and psychological symptoms (see Chapter 10).

There Are Many Available VR Apps in the Market; How Should I Choose?

It is recommended to choose VR content that is validated in scientific research in palliative care settings, ideally evidence-based, and validated by authorities such as the U.S. Food and Drug Administration.

How Can I Minimize Cybersickness Associated with VR Interventions?

To minimize the risks of cybersickness, VR facilitators can choose high-quality and high-resolution VR content and short VR durations. It is also recommended to screen out patients who are prone to motion sickness.

How Do I Resolve the Subjective Weight Issue of VR?

In addition to purchasing VR headsets that have lower objective weight, the VR facilitator or patient assistant can consider holding the VR headset when worn by patients.

How Do I Resolve the Visual Issue of VR?

Individual VR devices should have specific guidelines on how to adjust the VR headset for visual acuity. If the patient reports "image too blurred," adjustments should be made according to the guidelines. In addition, the visual issues may stem from the patient's visual limitations, such as short-sightedness, which may require wearing corrective glasses, and age-related issues, such as presbyopia or cataracts.

What Is the Best Time to Approach Patients for VR Interventions?

To minimize the physical burden on patients, it is advised to find the optimal time for VR sessions, such as the morning or before rehabilitation exercises, and to avoid times when patients are unwell or fatigued.

What Is the Best Environmental Condition for VR Interventions?

In a clinical setting, it is advised to use curtains for privacy and avoid disruptions. A quiet and safe environment is recommended for VR interventions.

What Is the Best Personnel Delivery for VR?

It is advised to have well-trained professionals for the ethical and quality delivery of VR interventions. Please refer to Chapter 12 for the knowledge, skills, and attitudes needed for qualified VR facilitators in palliative care.

How Do I Check if a Patient is Viewing Properly with the VR Headset?

An ideal condition is using a laptop or another device to have a real-time view of the patient's virtual environment. Without such a display, it is recommended to verbally check with patients about their experiences during VR exposure.

References

Beauchamp, T. L., & Childress, J. F. (2019). *Principles of biomedical ethics* (8th ed.). Oxford University Press.

Perna, L., Lund, S., White, N., & Minton, O. (2021). The potential of personalized virtual reality in palliative care: A feasibility trial. *American Journal of Hospice & Palliative Medicine, 38*(12), 1488–1494.

Saredakis, D., Szpak, A., Birckhead, B., Keage, H. A. D., Rizzo, A., & Loetscher, T. (2020). Factors associated with virtual reality sickness in head-mounted displays: A systematic review and meta-analysis. *Frontiers in Human Neuroscience, 14,* 96. https://doi.org/10.3389/fnhum.2020.00096

Weingarten, K., Macapagal, F., & Parker, D. (2020). Virtual reality: Endless potential in pediatric palliative care: A case report. *Journal of Palliative Medicine, 23*(1), 147–149. https://doi.org/10.1089/jpm.2019.0207

Wong, C. L., Li, C. K., Chan, C. W. H., Choi, K. C., Chen, J., Yeung, M. T., & Chan, O. N. (2021). Virtual reality intervention targeting pain and anxiety among pediatric cancer patients undergoing peripheral intravenous cannulation: A randomized controlled trial. *Cancer Nursing, 44*(6), 435–442. https://doi.org/10.1097/NCC.0000000000000844

15 Relevant Resources

This chapter highlights resources related to the use of virtual reality in palliative care, including relevant journals, international conferences, workshops, and potential networks for practitioners in this emergent clinical field. Despite the growing body of research on VR applications in healthcare, resources specifically targeting palliative care remain limited. This chapter aims to bridge that gap by providing information that, while primarily focused on palliative care, can also serve as valuable tools for presenting research findings and fostering connections among professionals with similar interests and expertise in VR practice. While this chapter presents a range of resources related to the use of virtual reality and palliative care, it is important to note that the list is not exhaustive. These suggestions serve as a starting point for researchers or practitioners seeking to expand their knowledge and networks in this emerging clinical field.

Journals Related to VR Research or Palliative Care

Journals	Main Theme	Links
Journal of Virtual Reality	VR	https://link.springer.com/journal/10055
Frontiers - **Frontiers in Virtual Reality** - **Frontiers in medical technology** - **Frontiers in digital health**	VR/digital health	https://www.frontiersin.org/journals/virtual-reality https://www.frontiersin.org/journals/medical-technology https://www.frontiersin.org/journals/digital-health
BMJ Open	Healthcare	https://bmjopen.bmj.com/
BMJ Supportive & Palliative Care	Palliative care	https://spcare.bmj.com/
Palliative Medicine	Palliative care	https://journals.sagepub.com/home/pmj

(Continued)

DOI: 10.4324/9781003518327-21

(Continued)

Journals	Main Theme	Links
Journal of Palliative Care	Palliative care	https://journals.sagepub.com/home/pala
American Journal of Hospice & Palliative Medicine	Palliative care	https://journals.sagepub.com/home/ajh
BMC Palliative Care	Palliative care	https://bmcpalliatcare.biomedcentral.com/

International Conferences or Workshop Related to VR Research or Palliative Care

International Conferences/Workshop	Link	Remarks
IEEE International Symposium on Mixed and Augmented Reality (ISMAR)	https://www.ismar.net/	The IEEE ISMAR is the leading international academic conference in the fields of Augmented Reality and Mixed Reality. The symposium is organized and supported by the IEEE Computer Society, IEEE VGTC, and ACM SIGCHI.
Virtual Reality and Healthcare Global Symposium	https://health24.ivrha.org/	The symposium is an annual event held by the International Virtual Reality and Healthcare Association (IVRHA), which aims at facilitating and supporting the growth of virtual reality in health and life sciences.
International Conference on Grief and Bereavement in Contemporary Society	https://www.socsc.hku.hk/icgb2014/	ICGB is a tri-annual event where global leaders in Thanatology and experts in various death-related disciplines meet to share their work and insights on issues of loss, trauma, and mortality.
World Research Congress of the European Association for Palliative Care	https://eapcnet.eu/ https://eapccongress.eu/2024/	The annual palliative care congress is held by the European Association for Palliative Care to support the promotion and development of palliative care throughout Europe and beyond.
The Annual Assembly of Hospice and Palliative Care	https://aahpm.org/	The annual Assembly is held by the American Academy of Hospice and Palliative Medicine to improve the care of patients and families with serious illnesses.

(Continued)

(Continued)

International Conferences/ Workshop	Link	Remarks
Asia Pacific Hospice Palliative Care Conference	https://www. aphc2025.com/	The biennial Asia Pacific Hospice Conferences of the Asia Pacific Hospice Palliative Care Network (APHN) were inaugurated in 1989 with the dual aims of enhancing our knowledge in hospice palliative care and networking within the region.
ISG World Conference on Gerontechnology	https://www. isg2024.com/ gb/	The conference is held by the International Society for Geotechnology (ISG) and takes place every two years, with a focus on reshaping ageing with technology.

Potential Network Related to Palliative Care

Potential network/association	
The Worldwide Hospice Palliative Care Alliance (WHPCA)	https://thewhpca.org/
Asia Pacific Hospice Palliative Care Network (APHN)	https://aphn.org/
European Association for Palliative Care (EAPC)	https://eapcnet.eu/
International Association for Hospice and Palliative Care (IAHPC)	https://hospicecare.com/home/
Palliative Care Network	https://palliativecarenetwork.com/
Australasian Palliative Link International	https://apli.net.au/
Association for Palliative Medicine of Great Britain and Ireland	https://apmonline.org/
American Academy of Hospice and Palliative Medicine	https://aahpm.org/

Epilogue

As I come to the end of this book, I want to express my heartfelt gratitude to you, my dear reader, for your interest and curiosity in exploring the therapeutic potential of VR for patients in need of palliative care. I commend your compassionate heart to help our vulnerable patients and your willingness to try novel interventions that can potentially make a meaningful difference in their lives. Writing this book has been a profound journey for me, one that has allowed me to share my clinical experiences and impart the knowledge I have gained over the years in this clinical field.

I humbly invite you to share what you have found most helpful to those who also have an interest in delivering VR interventions to patients with terminal illnesses. My dream is that all patients who may benefit from VR interventions can enjoy its magical power during the last journey of their lives. If you have any feedback and suggestions, please do not reserve sharing with me; it will help me make this book more useful and impactful for aspiring VR facilitators who are about to follow in your footsteps. If you have any suggestions or dislike any aspect of the book, please kindly let me know too. I value every comment from you.

Thank you once again for your time and interest. I look forward to connecting with you further through a newsletter, where I have been freely providing updated research on the evolving use of VR in palliative care. If you are interested in the newsletter, please reach out to me at olivewookitling@ gmail.com. Please join me in exploring the transformative power of VR and its ability to bring joy, comfort, and solace to those facing the most difficult moments of their lives.

I wish you peace, health, and happiness.

DOI: 10.4324/9781003518327-22

Index

Note: Page numbers in **bold** indicate a table on the corresponding page.